Contents

contents

INSTANT
DIET
MAKEOVER

- **Break Your Bad Habits**

- **Learn to Eat Smarter**

- **Lose Weight Quickly**

- **Keep It Off for a Lifetime**

ALEX A. LLUCH
Author of Over 3 Million Books Sold!

WS Publishing Group
San Diego, California 92119

INSTANT DIET MAKEOVER
By Alex A. Lluch

Published by WS Publishing Group
San Diego, California 92119
Copyright © 2010 by WS Publishing Group

Nutritional and fitness guidelines based on information provided by the United States Food and Drug Administration, Food and Nutrition Information Center, National Agricultural Library, Agricultural Research Service, and the U.S. Department of Agriculture.

Designed by: David Defenbaugh, WS Publishing Group

Image Credit: © iStockphoto

For inquiries:
Log on to www.WSPublishingGroup.com
E-mail info@WSPublishingGroup.com

ISBN-13: 978-1-936061-03-7

Printed in China

Introduction

Millions of people struggle with their weight every day. In the United States, the numbers of overweight adults has climbed to 67 percent, with 34 percent being considered obese. Anyone who is overweight knows about the myriad health problems this creates, from heart disease to diabetes to infertility to increased risk of cancer. Perhaps most tangible and immediate, however, are the feelings of sadness, failure and hopelessness that constantly battling your weight can cause. Like making any major lifestyle change, losing weight is a fight, so you must arm yourself with the most knowledge possible.

Instant Diet Makeover is here to give you that knowledge, to reveal the little white diet lies we tell ourselves that keep us from shedding pounds and inches. Are you relying on buzzwords like "organic" and "low-fat" to help you lose weight, but to no avail? Do you believe ordering a salad is enough of an effort to produce the results you want? Have you noticed that you often eat late at night, instead of when you're actually hungry, but don't know how to stop? Are you clueless as to why frozen diet meals aren't helping you slim down? These and many other common yet often-overlooked behaviors are featured in the chapters of this book, along with the information you need to break these bad diet habits, make permanent lifestyle changes and start losing weight.

This book helps you recognize where you've been fooling yourself and where you're completely clueless when it comes to food. Each section will have you gasping, "Wow, that's me! I can't believe I've been doing that!" while giving you the tools you need to remedy your bad habits. You'll learn to:

- Be completely honest with yourself about your bad diet habits
- Practice conscious eating
- Stop sabotaging your diet by making unhealthy tradeoffs
- Find easy places in your current diet to cut back on calories, fats, carbs, sodium and chemical additives
- Anticipate and recognize situations that cause you to overeat or eat unhealthy foods
- Pinpoint the emotions and triggers that cause you to overeat
- Develop a game plan for how to avoid pitfalls and stick to your healthy habits
- Determine the "diet" products that cause overeating

- Keep accountable for what you eat and drink by using a food diary
- Stop ruining healthy foods by eating them in unhealthy ways
- Identify common buzzwords that trick you into thinking you're eating healthy
- Recognize the changes you can make without starving or depriving yourself
- Develop new eating habits that will help you lose weight and that you can maintain for a lifetime!

It's time to get real about your bad diet habits and what changes it's going to take for you to lose weight. Whether you've been struggling with a lot of extra weight or just those frustrating last 10 pounds, you'll find yourself in the pages of this book, along with an array of permanent solutions to choose from. Discover what works for you on a long-term basis, since the goal of your weight-loss journey is to keep the weight off for good. No more rollercoaster dieting, which only saps your motivation and leads to sadness and frustration. You never have to give up on weight loss, you simply need to recognize where to change, adapt, and arm yourself with knowledge and insight.

Here's to eating smarter, being healthier, living longer and feeling better about yourself!

Your Health & Weight Status

You already know that you need and want to lose weight. The most important reasons to lose weight are to look and feel great and also to reduce the risk of health complications such as heart disease and diabetes.

Before you start using the secrets included in this book to make over your diet, it is important to assess your health status. There are three considerations when determining your current condition: your family history, waist size and Body Mass Index (BMI).

First, your personal history and family background can shed light on possible health risks. Be aware of increased potential problems if your family history includes arthritis, high blood pressure, high cholesterol, high blood sugar, death at a young age, heart problems, cancer, or respiratory illness. A history of family illness doesn't mean these conditions are destined to be a part of your future, but it is yet another reason to get started on the road to healthy eating and real lifestyle changes.

Now, use a tape measure to calculate your waist circumference below your rib cage and above your belly button. If your waist size is more than 35 inches for women and 40 inches for men, you have an increased health risk for developing serious chronic illness.

Body Mass Index - BMI

Body composition can vary greatly from individual to individual. Two people who possess the same height and weight can have different bone structure and varying percentages of muscle and fat. Therefore, your weight alone is not the only factor in assessing your risk for weight-related health issues. Your BMI can help indicate whether or not your health is at risk.

The first step is to measure your height and weight. You will need those two numbers to find your BMI. If your BMI falls within the range of 19 to 24, you are considered healthy. If your BMI lands from 25 to 29, then you have an increased risk of developing health problems. If your BMI is 30 or above, you could be considered obese.

Calculating your BMI: Locate your height in the left-hand column below. Then move across the row to your weight. The number at the very top of the column is your BMI.

BMI	19	20	21	22	23	24	25	26	27	28	29	30	31	32	33	34	35
Height							**Weight in pounds**										
4'10"	91	96	100	105	110	115	119	124	129	134	138	143	148	153	158	162	167
4'11"	94	99	104	109	114	119	124	128	133	138	143	148	153	158	163	168	173
5'	97	102	107	112	118	123	128	133	138	143	148	153	158	163	158	174	179
5'1"	100	106	111	116	122	127	132	137	143	148	153	158	164	169	174	180	185
5'2"	104	109	115	120	126	131	136	142	147	153	158	164	169	175	180	186	191
5'3"	107	113	118	124	130	135	141	146	152	158	163	169	175	180	186	191	197
5'4"	110	116	122	128	134	140	145	151	157	163	169	174	180	186	192	197	204
5'5"	114	120	126	132	138	144	150	156	162	168	174	180	186	192	198	204	210
5'6"	118	124	130	136	142	148	155	161	167	173	179	186	192	198	204	210	216
5'7"	121	127	134	140	146	153	159	166	172	178	185	191	198	204	211	217	223
5'8"	125	131	138	144	151	158	164	171	177	184	190	197	203	210	216	223	230
5'9"	128	135	142	149	155	162	169	176	182	189	196	203	209	216	223	230	236
5'10"	132	139	146	153	160	167	174	181	188	195	202	209	216	222	229	236	243
5'11"	136	143	150	157	165	172	179	186	193	200	208	215	222	229	236	243	250
6'	140	147	154	162	169	177	184	191	199	206	213	221	228	235	242	250	258
6'1"	144	151	159	166	174	182	189	197	204	212	219	227	235	242	250	257	265
6'2"	148	155	163	171	179	186	194	202	210	218	225	233	241	249	256	264	272
6'3"	152	160	168	176	184	192	200	208	216	224	232	240	248	256	264	272	279
	Healthy					**Overweight**						**Obese**					

Health Risks and Your Weight

For most adults, BMI and waist size are fairly reliable indicators of whether or not you are overweight. A higher waist size may indicate a greater risk for weight-related health issues such as high blood pressure, type-2 diabetes and coronary artery disease. Typically, the higher your Body Mass Index, the greater risk to your health. This risk also increases if your waist is greater than 35 inches for women or 40 inches for men.

If your weight indicates that you are at a higher risk for health problems, consult your primary care physician to determine safe and effective ways to improve your health. Even moderate amounts of weight loss, around 5 to 10 percent of your weight, can have long-lasting health benefits.

Risk of Associated Disease According to BMI and Waist Size

Body Mass Index		Waist less than or equal to 40" Men 35" Women	Waist greater than 40" Men 35" Women
18 or less	Underweight	N/A	N/A
19-24	Normal	N/A	N/A
25-29	Overweight	Increased	High
30-35	Obese	High	Very High
over 35	Obese	Very High	Very High

Secrets for Weight Loss

Daily Calories for Weight Maintenance

Your total daily calories should be based on your age, gender, body type, and level of physical activity. Active men should consume approximately 2,800 calories per day to maintain their ideal weight. Active women and sedentary men should eat 2,200 calories. Sedentary women and older adults should strive for 1,600 calories. If you are not sure how many daily calories you should consume, consult your primary care physician for a recommendation.

1,600 CALORIES

Sedentary women and older adults should consume approximately 1,600 calories daily.

2,200 CALORIES

Most children, teenage girls, active women and sedentary men should consume approximately 2,200 calories daily. Pregnant or breast-feeding women may need to consume more.

2,800 CALORIES

Most teenage boys and active men and some very active women should consume approximately 2,800 calories daily.

Suggested Daily Calories for Weight Loss

The total number of daily calories for a weight-loss plan will depend on the number of pounds you wish to lose. Once you have determined the daily number of calories that you should eat to maintain your weight, you should decrease your total caloric intake by an average of 500 calories per day for moderate weight loss. To proceed in a safe and healthy manner, you can eliminate those 500 calories simply by decreasing the amount of sugars, refined carbohydrates, and alcohol in your diet, most of which provide calories with little nutritional value.

Recommended Daily Amount from Each Food Group

The United States Department of Agriculture is known for its Food Guide, which is a nutritional reference for many health groups and dietary plans. The USDA Food Guide separates the foods you should eat into six different categories: 1) grains, 2) vegetables, 3) fruits, 4) fats and oils, 5) milk and dairy products, and 6) meat, beans, fish, and nuts. The suggested amounts below have been developed to help you select the proper amount of food to eat from each group on a daily basis. Each group provides you with a different set of essential nutrients. By following the recommended serving sizes, you can be assured that you are getting the proper amounts of protein, fats, carbohydrates, fiber, vitamins, and minerals. This guide can be adjusted to suit your personal needs and desired weight loss.

DAILY AMOUNT OF FOOD FROM EACH GROUP

Daily Calorie Level	1,200	1,400	1,600	1,800	2,000	2,200	2,400	2,600	2,800	3,000
Fruits	1 C (2 srv)	1.5 C (3 srv)	1.5 C (3 srv)	1.5 C (3 srv)	2 C (4 srv)	2 C (4 srv)	2 C (4 srv)	2 C (4 srv)	2.5 C (5 srv)	2.5 C (5 srv)
Vegetables	1.5 C (3 srv)	1.5 C (2 srv)	2 C (4 srv)	2.5 C (5 srv)	2.5 C (5 srv)	3 C (6 srv)	3 C (6 srv)	3.5 C (7 srv)	3.5 C (7 srv)	4 C (8 srv)
Grains	4 oz.	5 oz.	5 oz.	6 oz.	6 oz.	7 oz.	8 oz	9 oz.	10 oz.	10 oz.
Meat, Beans, Fish & Nuts	3 oz.	4 oz.	5 oz.	5 oz.	5.5 oz.	6 oz.	6.5 oz.	6.5 oz.	7 oz.	7 oz
Milk	2 C	2 C	3 C	3 C	3 C	3 C	3 C	3 C	3 C	3 C
Fats & Oils	17 g	17 g	22 g	24 g	27 g	29 g	31 g	34 g	36 g	44 g
Food Group	Food group amounts shown in cups (C) or ounces (oz.), with number of servings (srv) in parentheses. Oils are shown in grams.									

The Benefit of Drinking Water

Drinking eight 8-ounce glasses of water each day is an excellent addition to your routine. Try drinking a glass before and during each meal to promote feeling full and therefore encouraging the body to eat less. Sometimes a feeling of hunger, along with fatigue or headaches, is actually a sign of dehydration. The average adult loses over 2 quarts of water each day. Once your body sends you a message that it is thirsty, you are already dehydrated.

Not only will drinking water at regular intervals keep you hydrated, it can also help you keep your calories down. If you can get used to drinking water at meals instead of a 20-ounce bottle of soda or an alcoholic beverage, you can reduce approximately 250 calories at each meal.

A Breakdown of the Nutritional Facts Label

When you're on a weight-loss and diet plan, you need to know how to read the nutritional facts label for the ingredient list, serving size, calories, amounts, nutrients, portions, and percentage of daily nutritional values.

All Calories Are Not Created Equal: Calories provide a concrete measure of how much energy you receive from a serving size of a selected food. You should also be aware of how many calories per serving come from fat. Let's say there are 250 calories in a serving, and 110 of those come from fat. That means almost half of the calories are from fat. To lose weight, select foods with 20 percent or less of its calories per serving coming from fat. These can be from proteins, dairy products, and whole grain breads, cereals, pasta, and fresh fruits and vegetables.

Keep Tabs on Cholesterol: Cholesterol is a fat-like substance present in all animal foods, such as meat, poultry, fish, milk and milk products, and egg yolks. Eating foods high in dietary cholesterol increases the risk of heart disease. Most health authorities suggest dietary cholesterol should be limited to 300 mg or less per day. Select lean meats, avoid eating the skin of poultry, and use low-fat milk products.

Salt and Sodium: It's important to include some salt in your diet, but it should be limited to 2,400 mg per day. Go easy on luncheon and cured meats, cheeses, canned soups and vegetables, and soy sauce. Look for no-salt-added products at your supermarket. Be cautious and avoid adding table salt to your food. Each teaspoon of salt adds 2,000 mg of sodium to your diet. So put down the salt shaker and retrain your taste buds.

Sugar, How Sweet It Isn't: Here's a list of common sweeteners that are essentially sugar: white sugar, honey, sucrose, fructose, maltose, lactose, syrup, corn syrup, high fructose corn syrup, molasses, and fruit juice concentrate. If these terms are found in the first four listings on the label, that food is likely to be very high in sugar.

Consider that 4 grams are to equal 1 teaspoon of sugar. The total daily intake for all added sugar sources not found naturally in the food itself should be a maximum 6 teaspoons a day.

Carbohydrates: Breads, cereals, rice, and pasta provide carbohydrates, which are excellent sources of energy. Although you are on a weight-loss plan, it is important to include them in your diet because they provide vitamins, minerals, and fiber. One serving of carbohydrates equals one slice of bread, one ounce of ready-to-eat cereal, or 1/2 cup cooked cereal, rice or pasta. Focus on complex carbohydrates, such as whole grain breads, cereals, and brown rice. Keep these foods healthy by not adding additional butter, margarine, cream, cheese, sugar, oils, and fat. Limit refined carbohydrates, such as white flour and sugar, as well as processed foods like prepackaged candy, cookies, cakes, and chips.

Fruits & Vegetables: Eat a rainbow of fruits and vegetables to lose weight and stay full. For example, eat a yellow banana, green broccoli, orange carrots, a red apple, purple cabbage, and blueberries. Fruits and vegetables provide vitamins A and C, and folate. They also contain minerals like iron, potassium, and magnesium. Keep in mind that it is important to eat these foods as fresh as possible, preferably raw. When you can, choose the actual piece of fruit, like an apple, over juice.

Protein: The USDA Food Guide suggests eating cooked lean meat as a source of protein for optimum health. Protein provides an essential supply of B vitamins, zinc, and iron. Make sure you get enough of these nutrients by combining a variety of choices, such as lean cuts of beef, pork, veal, lamb, chicken, turkey, fish, and shellfish. Other protein possibilities are eggs, beans, nut butters, tofu, dried nuts, and seeds. Try to choose lean cuts of meat, remove the skin from poultry, trim away all visible fat, go easy on egg yolks, and eat nuts and seeds sparingly.

Fat: As a food source, fat supplies energy and essential fatty acids to your body. Fat-soluble vitamins like A, D, E and K and carotenoids need fat to be absorbed into the body. Not all types of fat are healthy, however, especially saturated fats found in whole milk, butter, ice cream, poultry skin, and palm oil. Unsaturated fats, found mainly in vegetable oils, do not increase blood cholesterol.

A third category called trans fat is formed when liquid oils are made into solid fats, like shortening and hard margarine. This type of fat is dangerous because it raises blood cholesterol and increases the risk of coronary heart disease, which is one of the leading causes of death in the United States. Foods high in trans fat are processed foods made with partially hydrogenated vegetable oils, such as vegetable shortenings. These oils can be found in crackers, cookies, candies, snack foods, fried foods, and baked goods. It is difficult to avoid all foods with trans fat, so the ideal goal would be to limit your intake of processed foods as much as possible.

Healthy Fats: Try choosing vegetable oils like olive, canola, soybean, sunflower, and corn. Avoid coconut and palm kernel oils. Consider adding fish to your menu twice a week. Salmon and mackerel have omega-3 fatty acids, which offer protection against heart disease. Choose lean meats like skinless chicken, lean beef, and pork.

Best Sources for Essential Nutrients

Best Sources of Calcium
Milk and dairy: yogurt, cheese, milk
Seafood: sardines, pink salmon, perch, blue crab, clams
Various vegetables: collard, turnip, and dandelion greens, spinach
Peas/beans/legumes: soybeans/tofu, black-eyed peas, white beans
Fortified foods: cereals, soy milk, oatmeal

Best Sources of Iron
Shellfish: clams, oysters, shrimp
Organ meats: liver, giblets
Beans/legumes/peas: soy, white, kidney, lima, navy, lentils
Lean meats: beef, duck, lamb
Various fruit/vegetables: spinach, prune juice, tomato puree/paste

Best Sources of B Vitamins
Organ meats: liver
Lean protein: pork, poultry, eggs, fish
Whole grains: brown rice, whole wheat bread, oatmeal
Legumes/nuts: soy beans, peanuts, walnuts

Best Sources of Vitamin A
Organ meats: liver, giblets
Dark leafy vegetables: collard, turnip, and mustard greens, kale
Orange fruit/vegetables: carrots, sweet potato, pumpkin, squash

Best Sources of Vitamin C
Various fruits: guava, kiwi, orange, grapefruit, strawberries, cantaloupe, papaya, pineapple, mango
Various vegetables: red/green sweet pepper, brussels

sprouts, broccoli, sweet potato, cauliflower, kale

Best Sources of Vitamin E
Fortified foods: ready-to-eat cereals
Seeds & nuts: sunflower seeds, almonds, pine nuts, hazelnuts
Oils: sunflower, cottonseed, safflower, canola, peanut

Best Sources of Potassium
Various vegetables: sweet potato, tomato puree/paste, beet greens, potato, carrot juice, winter squash, spinach
Beans/legumes/peas: white beans, soybeans, lentils, kidney beans
Milk & dairy: yogurt, milk
Various fruits: prune juice, bananas, peaches, prunes, apricots

Chapter 1

Eating Foods Unhea

Healthy
in
Healthy Ways

Eating Healthy Foods in Unhealthy Ways

Ever since you first learned about the food pyramid when you were a child, you have had an idea of the foods that are healthier for you, including fruits, vegetables and whole grains. However, what you eat doesn't matter if you don't consider how you prepare and order it, and too many dieters fool themselves into thinking ordering a side of vegetables or a salad is enough of an effort.

Losing weight takes knowledge and dedication, and you have to be aware of the ways in which healthy foods are made in unhealthy ways.

For instance, one in five Americans say they eat salad every day or every other day, but while salad appears to be the golden ticket of dieting, it can quickly be made into a 1,000-calorie meal with a sprinkling of calorie-filled toppings. Restaurant salads are notoriously dangerous — portions are unreasonable and often include fried or cheesy additions. This chapter will give you an easy guide to choosing a salad — what to look for, what to avoid, and what toppings make for great taste without the added fat and calories.

Vegetables, in general, give dieters the impression they're eating healthy, although, like anything, they can be made in an abundance of unhealthy ways. Even raw veggies can turn into bite-size diet busters, depending on what you're dipping them into. Read on and you'll learn to spot the red flags that ruin low-calorie, nutrient-packed vegetables, as well as how to prepare dishes that keep veggies delicious and diet-friendly.

You'll also get real about the ways you may be sabotaging convenient, portion-controlled frozen diet meals by adding unhealthy extras or removing the very elements that give them their weight-loss benefits. This is one of those bad behaviors that is easy to overlook.

Finally, you'll learn to spot how your morning pick-me-up could be sabotaging your diet. Coffee can be a helpful diet tool as it suppresses hunger and kick-starts the metabolism for many people; however, it's an easy place for sneaky calories to throw off your entire day. On the flip side, this is an easy place to cut back and instantly eliminate tons of calories, fats and sugars.

You're not doing yourself any favors if you're eating healthy foods in unhealthy ways. Read on to make the changes it takes to start dropping pounds.

Instant Diet Makeover Tips:

▸ Don't be afraid to ask your server how the meal is prepared, or to request that the food be prepared in a way that is in line with your diet program.

▸ If you're having a cookout or barbecue, choose lean cuts of meat that have less fat or trim off excess fat before cooking.

▸ Fill up on low-density, high-volume foods, such as fruits, vegetables, soups and stews, cooked grains, lean meats, fish, and lean poultry.

▸ If you have diabetes, food allergies, or are a vegetarian, consult a dietetics professional on how you can safely lose weight.

▸ Eating fish is a good way to increase the healthy fats in your diet, which can help reduce the risk of heart attacks.

▸ Tofu is a good substitute for many foods because it is rich in high-quality protein and contains no cholesterol. Try using it in place of cream in sauces.

▸ Remember that small measurable steps toward weight loss are often the most gratifying!

Salad Sabotage!

The Misconception:

You're most likely one of the 70 to 80 percent of Americans who eat salad at least once a week, possibly part of the 21 percent who say they eat a salad every day or almost every day. You enjoy salads on the side of many meals and often have a large green salad for lunch or dinner. You buy a crisp head of iceberg lettuce and pile on the toppings, such as crunchy croutons, bacon, hardboiled eggs, cranberries, ham, shredded cheese and more. Like most Americans, your favorite dressings are probably Ranch and blue cheese. If you're having pasta for dinner, you might whip up a tasty Caesar salad. When you get sick of field greens, you like to pick up convenient ready-made side salads from the grocery store deli, such as potato salad, pasta salad or broccoli salad. To cut calories, you look to order a salad when you eat out at restaurants; for example, you'll order a taco salad when you go out for Mexican food.

Well, unfortunately, the simple act of ordering a salad doesn't a healthy meal make. Stop pretending that the word "salad" automatically means healthy or that it represents the holy grail of dieting. A salad clad in the wrong dressings or toppings can actually have more calories and fat than a hamburger and fries or a plate of creamy pasta.

Your first and most obvious mistake is your dressing choice. A study of 1,000 people by Kraft Foods found that the top choices of salad dressing for women were Ranch, 33 percent; blue cheese, 12 percent; vinaigrette, 11 percent; Italian, 9 percent; and French/Catalina, 7 percent. Men's top choices were Ranch, 27 percent; blue cheese, 15 percent; French/Catalina, 11 percent; Thousand Island, 10 percent; and Italian, 10 percent. Clearly, creamy dressings are the favorites of both men and women. They are also the quickest way to turn your healthy meal into salad sabotage.

The culprit here is mayonnaise, which is the main ingredient that gives Ranch, blue cheese, Thousand Island, Caesar and other smooth dressings their creaminess. Full-fat mayo boasts nearly 100 calories per tablespoon, rendering these dressings completely useless for anyone trying to lose weight. Just two tablespoons of Ranch dressing (and you probably use much more than that on a large salad — don't lie) have 150 calories and 25 percent of your daily value of fat. Do yourself a favor and eliminate these dressings from your repertoire, immediately. You are now wearing creamy salad dressing blinders, people!

Also beware of vinaigrettes that load up with sugar to achieve better taste. Check labels and use them sparingly when dining out.

The second, only slightly less obvious evil-doers are the toppings you're choosing. When you pile on oily, fatty toppings — bacon bits, fried chicken (ack!), cheese, croutons — you're also piling on the calories and saturated fat. Fruit and nuts are also a fast way for hundreds of extra calories to sneak into your leafy greens. A too-bland salad will always disappoint and leave you hungry for a snack an hour later, just be smarter when choosing protein and toppings.

> Stop pretending that the word "salad" automatically means healthy or that it represents the holy grail of dieting.

That brings us to the lettuce. Iceberg lettuce might have a nice crunch, but it's worthless nutritionally. Anything is better, but the darker the leaves the more nutrients they pack.

Now, let's chat about deli-aisle salads. In general, these are a big, fat mistake. Typical grocery story choices — English pea, pasta, potato, Waldorf, macaroni, broccoli, chicken, tuna and egg salads — are all full of mayo. It's what holds these salads together, giving them their consistency. These are not healthy sides. These are not "salads" like you want them to be — "salads" meaning fresh, healthy and satisfying.

Your salad shouldn't come in a bowl the size of a wok.

Now let's talk about the taco salad. Suffice to say that any salad that comes in a deep-fried shell is not a dieters' salad. Remove the unhealthy parts of a taco salad — the shell, the sour cream, the cheese and the refried beans — and you're left with little resembling Mexican cuisine. Remember that the word salad doesn't automatically give something license to help you lose weight. Restaurants, with their 1,100-calorie entrée salads, proved this point long ago.

The Way to Lose Weight:

Salads can, of course, be one of your best weight-loss friends. Frequently eating green salads with raw veggies means your body will be getting crucial nutrients and antioxidants, such as vitamins A, C and E, folic acid, fiber, lycopene, and beta-carotene.

A great diet trick is eating a small green salad before your meal. Research has shown that eating a green salad of 150 calories or less reduces the total number of calories eaten during the meal and helps you feel full and satisfied.

When you're making salads as lunch or dinner, you'll want to eat a large enough portion to satiate you, but without weighing it down with calories and fat.

Here are your salad rules for weight loss:

- Top your salad with lean, clean protein (chicken, portabello mushrooms, lean strip steak, seared ahi), not mayo-rich egg, chicken or tuna salad.

- Fried chicken, fried onion strings, crunchy noodles and fried wonton strips are out! These items do not come on a real salad! Don't be ridiculous.

- You can't have bacon, cheese *and* croutons. Choose one. Use it sparingly. And you can always make a healthier choice when it comes to cheese. Low-fat mozzarella sticks can be shredded onto a salad or sprinkle a small amount of feta cheese — a little gives a lot of flavor and it is naturally lower in fat and calories than others.

- Ready-made grocery store salads are almost always a no. Most are packed with gooey, fat-filled mayo. A better choice that you can make on your own in a hurry: fruit salad. Chop a banana, apple and red grapes and add a can of drained mandarin oranges. Sprinkle cinnamon over the top and you have enough to feed two to four people a sweet side salad with no fat and only natural sugars. Another healthier, lighter option is to make tuna salad Mediterranean style, with chopped celery, olives, olive oil, lemon juice, and salt and pepper.

- Dressing on the side, always. Don't ever trust restaurant dressings! Even the light-sounding dressings on the menu, such as raspberry vinaigrette or Asian sesame vinaigrette, for instance, are full of sugar. And restaurants are infamous for pouring on far too much dressing. A weight-loss tip: Dip your fork into the dressing cup several times and spread it over the salad. You'll get the flavor of the dressing without soaking your salad and adding calories.

- Ask for oil and vinegar if available. A few splashes of red wine or balsamic vinegar are often all you need on a vegetable salad.

- No taco shells! No tostada salads! None! If you want south-of-the-border flavor in a salad, combine romaine lettuce hearts, low-sodium black beans, a sprinkle of pepper jack cheese, chunks of avocado and salsa. Add red pepper strips and a few black olives too, if you like.

- Your salad shouldn't come in a bowl the size of a wok. Restaurants are notorious for offering larger-than-life salads. But many also offer "appetizer-size" or "lunch portion" salads. Opt for those. If you do order a salad that is huge, put dressing only on half and take the other half home. Eat it in the next day so it's still crisp.

- Studies have shown that people associate crunch with satisfaction and satiation. No, bacon does not count as a viable crunchy topping. Think water chestnuts, cucumbers, grapes, non-candied nuts, bell peppers, cauliflower, apples and pears.

- Sorry, but Caesar is a no. It doesn't generally include much more than cheesy croutons and shaved parmesan. And the main ingredients in creamy Caesar dressing are mayo, oil and eggs. Yuck.

- Iceberg lettuce lacks any real nutritional value. Choose a darker lettuce like spring greens, arugula, or spinach. To achieve the same crunch as iceberg with several times as many nutrients, romaine is a good choice.

Veggies on the Side Can't Be Buttered or Fried

The Misconception:

When dining out, your entrée comes with a choice of side dish, including fries, rice, or vegetables. Easy, right? Pass on the French fries, order the veggies, and pat yourself on the back. It is a mistake to think your work is done here, and an easy one to make. You assume the eatery is offering you vegetables as a "healthy" side dish option, but recognize that how the veggies are cooked and seasoned dictates how much they're going to aid in (or detract from) your weight loss.

Unfortunately, the easiest way for restaurants to cook typical side-dish veggies like zucchini, carrots, and broccoli to taste great is to sauté them in butter and salt. It's a bad sign when vegetables come served on a small side plate— they're probably soaking in butter. The extra plate keeps the melted butter-runoff contained and separate from your main meal.

Depending on what part of the country you're in a side

of vegetables may also mean — gasp — a trip to the deep fryer. Southern cooking, especially, has a penchant for deep-fried everything, from green beans to zucchini to tomatoes. Not for the faint of heart, and definitely not for anyone trying to lose weight.

Don't make the mistake of thinking just because you asked for a side of vegetables that you're making a healthy choice. Veggies bathed in butter or battered and fried mean hundreds of extra calories and tons of saturated fat.

When vegetables come served on a small side plate that's always a bad sign that they're soaking in butter.

The Way to Lose Weight:

Always inquire about how food is prepared when you eat out; it can save you hundreds of calories. Vegetable sides shouldn't be sautéed in butter, battered or deep-fried. Don't even accept "lightly dusted"! To keep them healthy and delicious, ask for your veggies steamed, sautéed in a touch of olive oil, or roasted. Don't feel guilty about sending them back if they come prepared in an unhealthy way! This defeats the purpose of ordering veggies — you may as well get the fries!

When you make them at home, try a splash of lemon juice, a drizzle of balsamic vinegar or a twist of black pepper before oven-baking vegetables like cauliflower or sweet potatoes.

Leave out the pads of butter from recipes like curried carrots — the rich spices already give the carrots a great flavor without the added calories and saturated fat.

Experiment and you'll find that many vegetables, like tomatoes and bell peppers, are delicious when baked or blackened on a grill, without adding much of anything. Remember, the fewer ingredients the better when it comes to keeping vegetables low-fat and low-calorie.

Don't give yourself a high five for choosing veggies over fries unless you're going to be sure they're cooked the right way!

Do You Know What's in Your Daily Latte?

The Misconception:

You feel good about your daily stop at the coffee shop, because you never order those sugary, whipped cream-topped drinks some people like. No chocolate shavings for you — you stick to a vanilla latte or a light frappuccino.

Aside from the fact that a medium or grande-size coffee drink is costing you between $2.50 and $4 a day, do you really know how many calories are in your morning pick-me-up? Unless you specify, coffee drinks are made with 2% milk, which adds fat, calories and carbs to your beverage. Additionally, any sweetener, such as flavored syrups, caramel, or cocoa powder, add dozens of calories and carbs as well.

You might not be surprised that a Grande Caramel Brulee Frappuccino from Starbucks boasts a whopping 300 calories, even without whipped cream, but did you realize that your standard vanilla latte has 250 calories, 4 grams of saturated fat, and 36 carbohydrates? Even "light" and "skinny" drinks add up to nearly 200 calories. And don't even get started on those seasonal drinks — the pumpkin and gingerbread lattes are like desserts in a cup.

> Looking for an effortless place to trim 200, 300, even 400 calories? Start at your neighborhood coffee shop.

The bottom line is this: The difference between your current weight and losing 10 pounds or more may be a matter of a few hundred calories. Looking for an effortless place to trim 200, 300, even 400 calories? Start at your neighborhood coffee shop. Even if you can't give up your caffeine habit, there are plenty of alternatives and modifications you can make that don't include sabotaging your diet with one little drink.

The Way to Lose Weight:

The upside of a coffee-and-milk-blended drink is the calcium and nutrients, which another caffeinated beverage, like a soda, won't provide. However, green or black tea, great alternatives to coffee, are full of disease-fighting antioxidants, offer a boost of caffeine, and have been shown to suppress appetite and aid in weight loss. With about 10 times the amount of antioxidants found in fruits and veggies, green and black teas have been widely used in traditional Asian medicine for centuries and are said to prevent everything from headaches to cancer.

If you can't live without coffee, the key to losing weight is to go as bare-bones as possible with your selections. Start with hot or iced Café Americano (aka, regular coffee). Sounds dull? It doesn't have to be! One or two pumps of sugar-free flavored syrup can jazz it up. If you must have milk, always ask for nonfat milk. And, cinnamon is a favorite coffee condiment of many dieters. It packs lots of flavor without the added sugar. Making this switch will let you start your day with under 25 calories per medium coffee.

A simple and delicious cup of brewed coffee can easily be your morning staple and a perfect place to eliminate a few hundreds calories, right from the start of your day.

Quit Picking at Your Healthy Prepackaged Meals

The Misconception:

When you peruse the frozen dinners section at the grocery store, you probably know to avoid the Salisbury steak or meat lasagna. Unfortunately, frozen green beans may not be your thing. Or maybe you wish the vegetarian enchiladas had just a little more cheese on top.

It's true that some prepackaged dinners don't look very appealing with their compartmentalized cardboard trays and pouches of sauce, thus many dieters admit to making a few "adjustments" to their frozen meals. If you're adding shredded cheese or guacamole to your low-fat frozen burrito, don't pretend you can keep the calorie count the same! The same goes for any extra sauces you add. Soy sauce, teriyaki, marinara and barbecue sauce all add calories, sodium and carbs.

Or are you picking the veggies out of your Lean Cuisine? Then the meal isn't providing the fiber and nutrients you need to feel satiated and lose weight. Without that serving of vegetables, you've taken an already-small meal down another notch. Odds are you'll be clamoring for a snack shortly after eating.

A main benefit of these meals is that they are portion-controlled and provide an accurate idea of how much fat, carbs, sodium and calories you're eating. This flies out the window when you alter the contents!

It's a common white lie that dieters tell themselves — they choose to ignore the calories that sneak in through extra sauces, dressings and toppings. If you're keeping a food diary

Don't do yourself a disservice by poking and prodding until you've eliminated all their health and weight-loss benefits.

(which you should be, hello!) you can't let these extras slide. The only way to lose weight is to have a true picture of what you're eating and drinking so you can see where to cut back.

The other benefit of frozen diet meals is that they are nutritionally balanced. Everything you need to lose weight in a healthy, smart way is right there in a convenient package. So don't make things complicated by removing the good stuff, like the vegetables. Duh!

The next time you're tempted to pick off the mushrooms or grate extra cheese over the top of your frozen flatbread pizza, ask yourself if the additional calories and lost nutrients are really worth it. You're messing with the calorie-controlled, nutritiously sound nature of the meal — and isn't that reason you shelled out $4 for that frozen dinner in the first place?

The Way to Lose Weight:

> Each component of the frozen meal is there for a reason — to create a portion that is sufficiently satisfying.

Frozen diet meals are generally about 6 ounces — not much to begin with. Don't do yourself a disservice by poking and prodding until you've eliminated all their health and weight-loss benefits. The only things you should be adding to your frozen meals are a side salad, a small whole-grain roll, an additional helping of vegetables, or a super-low-calorie topping like hot sauce or salsa.

And don't remove anything either! There are dozens of brands of diet meals, each offering literally hundreds of choices for flavor and cuisine. The days of sad-sack chicken breast and soggy broccoli are over! Now you can get everything from vegetarian to Mexican to pizza to Indian food in healthy, portion-controlled meals. This means you should have no problem finding a handful of choices where you enjoy every part of them.

Don't even skip the "dessert" portion that some meals offer, such as baked apples. You might think you're saving calories, but each component of the frozen meal is there for a reason — to create a portion large and satisfying enough that you won't need to eat anything additional afterward.

Another way to put your frozen dinners to work for weight loss: Save a few of the empty containers when you're done eating. Wash them out and use them as a model for proper portion sizes the next time you cook. Frozen diet meals can be an excellent teacher for understanding the right ratios of protein to vegetables to starch to sauce.

Whatever you do, don't sabotage your prepackaged meals. They have their place in your diet plan if you choose wisely and enjoy them the right way.

Don't Dip Into
Fat and Calories

The Misconception:

Cocktail parties, sports tailgates and get-togethers with friends call for snacks, and hors d'oeuvres and dips are an ever-popular option. From a gourmet spinach and artichoke dip to a spicy cheese dip to a creamy onion dip to a multi-layer bean dip, you take a dollop of each. Because you also load your plate with carrots, tomatoes, celery sticks and other vegetables, you assume you're enjoying a healthy snack. By eating all these veggies, you figure you'll eat less of the unhealthy burgers and bacon-wrapped weenies.

You're being fooled by the visual of a few spoonfuls of dip — their small size and consistency belie the fact that they pack a serious punch when it comes to fat and calories. Most of the most popular party dips are the creamy and cheesy versions, which have 200 calories or more per ¼-cup serving, more than 10 grams of fat, and include several grams of saturated fat. Ugh. Knowing that will spoil your appetite.

The other real issue here is that you're using these dips as a starter and planning to have other larger food items later. If you don't want to wreck your diet, you need a better game plan.

> Sour cream, cream cheese and mayo are the big three to avoid.

The Way to Lose Weight:

Remind yourself again and again: You can't go into any event — a pre-game tailgate or a friend's housewarming party — with no options. You never know what the host will provide, so you should bring something healthy so you'll have at least one low-calorie, low-fat choice, no matter what.

Skip the veggie tray from the grocery store, which almost always includes Ranch dressing. Buy veggies individually (usually cheaper than the pre-made tray anyhow), such as grape tomatoes, celery sticks, bell peppers, cauliflower and snap peas, and make your own healthy dip. A great one, even for the cooking-challenged, is hummus, which is just chickpeas, olive oil, tahini, lemon juice, garlic, and black and cayenne pepper blended to a smooth texture in a food processor. Or take another cue from the Greeks and buy garlic and cucumber tzatziki, which tastes delicious on vegetables and salads and is low-calorie and low-fat without losing any of the creaminess.

> You never know what the host will provide, so bring something healthy to have at least one low-calorie, low-fat choice.

This brings us to a great diet secret: Using Greek or other non-fat yogurt as a substitute for sour cream and mayo. You won't lose any of the creaminess of your favorite dips but with zero grams of fat and packed with protein, you're making a smart tradeoff.

Here's the good, the bad and the ugly of dips to help you stay on track with your daily calorie and fat intake:

Good:

- **Hummus:** Natural ingredients, low-calorie and plenty of varieties (roasted garlic, red pepper, spicy) make this a great choice.

- **Tzatziki:** Creamy but low-fat and very versatile

- **Eggplant dip:** Add a little cumin and green onion and this is a tasty low-fat dip you can make easily at home.

- **Dill-yogurt dip:** Made with Greek yogurt instead of sour cream, of course, with dill to pack a flavor punch

- **Curry dip:** Smooth over the exotic taste of curry and chili powder with low-fat yogurt and low-fat mayo for creaminess — without overloading the fat content

- **Salsa:** Super low-calorie and no fat, just watch the chips. Try toasted pita triangles instead.

- **Mediterranean layered dip:** A perfect substitute for layered bean dip (see the "Ugly" category), you can stack low-fat Greek yogurt, kalamata olives, feta, tomatoes, red pepper, cucumbers, garlic and whatever else you like. Top with chopped romaine lettuce and sprinkle paprika over the top.

- **Caviar:** Partying with the highbrow? If the host serves caviar, this is a low-calorie option you can enjoy without feeling guilty.

Bad:

- **Ranch or blue cheese:** By now, this should be a "duh" moment

- **French onion dip:** Sour cream, cream cheese and mayo are the big three to avoid, and this dip tends to have 'em all.

- **Cheese dip:** Includes tons of calories and fat — even more if it's made with ground beef, which is included in many warm varieties

- **Avocado dip:** Guacamole, when it's made with all-natural ingredients, contains good fats, but its cousin, avocado dip, has sour cream for smoothness and boasts more than 150 calories per serving.

- **Aioli or remoulade:** Honestly, these are just French for "mayonnaise" with a few spices. Watch out for them served as dipping sauces for seafood or steamed artichokes.

- **Any dip that comes in a can:** Prepackaged dips contain tons of sodium, preservatives and other unfortunate ingredients. Many are easy to make at home, so stay away from canned dips.

Ugly:

- **Spinach and artichoke dip:** Cheese and mayo make this a calorie explosion, especially since it tastes too good to stop at one bite.

- **Mexican bean dip:** Five layers, seven layers, whatever. Sour cream, refried beans, cheese and guacamole mean it's all bad.

- **Crab or seafood dip:** Mayo, cheese, cream cheese and fake seafood? You're looking at 300 calories or more per serving. A word to the wise: Avoid anything that comes in a bread bowl!

- **Bacon dip:** Salty bacon, cheese or cream cheese, jalapeños? Yikes! Full of fat, plus can you say, heartburn?

- **Fondue:** Cheese or chocolate fondue are two to stay far, far away from. Because you can't really scoop them onto your plate, it's nearly impossible to gauge how much you've eaten. Once again, when it's too good to stop, you should steer clear.

Tradec
Are Mc
You Fa

fs That

king

Tradeoffs That Are Making You Fat

A tradeoff, by definition, is giving up A in order to gain B. When it comes to losing weight, tradeoffs are one of the most important things smart dieters do for themselves.

Dieters recognize that giving up desserts in favor of fruit, for instance, can help them drop unwanted pounds quickly. Or they recognize that eating out less and cooking at home more — although eating out may be more fun — saves hundreds of calories at each meal. In weight loss, tradeoffs usually mean giving up something you enjoy for something less instantly gratifying but healthier in the long run. Diet tradeoffs are worth it because reaching an ideal weight, feeling great and being healthier are the ultimate payoffs.

However, there are some tradeoffs that are actually keeping you from losing weight. This is because too many dieters lie to themselves and believe that minimal effort in one area will lead to great weight-loss results. Unfortunately, that just isn't realistic. If losing weight were that easy, everyone would be thin and happy — 134 million Americans wouldn't be overweight.

This chapter will highlight a few of these unhealthy tradeoffs, such as saving calories in one area only to spend them in another, believing that vitamins will counteract an unhealthy lifestyle, or cooking at home only to snack and overeat throughout the process. Each tradeoff begins with a smart decision — swapping diet soda for full-sugar soda, cooking for yourself, or taking the stairs — but ends with a foolish decision that negates the benefits of the tradeoff. Not only are these tradeoffs useless but they're actually contributing to your inability to lose weight and packing on pounds.

In this chapter, you'll learn to recognize the mindsets that lead to weight gain — passiveness, complacency and ignorance. The wonderful thing is, once you stop these bad behaviors and start losing weight, you'll be filled with a new energy that will propel you to your new, healthier lifestyle. Nothing will be more motivating than recognizing bad habits, beginning new ones, and seeing the unwanted pounds come off!

Mark Twain once joked, "The only way to keep your health is to eat what you don't want, drink what you don't like, and do what you'd rather not." But this doesn't have to be true! Being healthy and getting to the weight you want is really all about moderation, planning ahead, and making smart tradeoffs that have *real* benefits to you.

Instant Diet Makeover Tips:

▶ Set temporary or short-term goals for yourself. Breaking the journey down into smaller sections can make it easier to stay on track.

▶ Get moving: An active person burns approximately 30 percent of their calories through daily non-exercise activity, versus 15 percent for sedentary people.

▶ Beware: Caffeine can give you that boost you need to wake up in the morning but it can also trick your body into thinking it's hungry when it's not.

▶ Make a list of all the foods you like that fit within your diet program so you can easily plan meals and grocery lists.

▶ Chicken broth and fresh herbs are an excellent and delicious substitute for butter and margarine when cooking.

▶ If you can't make it to the gym every day, try to incorporate other physical activities into your day, such as gardening, vacuuming or even shopping.

▶ Stay motivated by documenting changes to your weight, body size, energy and mood on a weekly and monthly basis.

Diet Soda Can Lead to More Calories

The Misconception:

You've given up full-sugar soda in favor of Diet Coke — good job, right? Wrong. Actually, studies have consistently linked diet soda intake with being overweight and obese. In fact, eight years of data studied by Sharon P. Fowler and her colleagues at the University of Texas Health Science Center in San Antonio found that for each can of diet soft drink consumed each day, a person's risk of obesity went up by 41 percent.

For one, diet soda has zero nutritional value, so the notion that you're doing something good for yourself is nonsense. Soda contains no nutrients, although it is ultra-acidic, about the same pH as vinegar, with sugar or aspartame used to mask the acidity. And, when you drink one or more diet sodas a day, you're not making room for drinks that do have nutritional value, like juice or tea.

But more significantly, diet soda can actually make you want to eat more! Aspartame, which replaces real sugar in diet soft drinks, is actually about 200 times sweeter than sugar. That artificial sweet taste triggers the pleasure centers in your brain, but without delivering an influx of calories, making you actually crave more calories afterward. Fowler explains that the body "will search for the calories promised but not delivered." In fact, a Purdue University study published in the *International Journal of Obesity* found that rats that were fed artificial sweeteners ate three times more high-calorie food than the rats that were fed real sugar. Many researchers believe that, over time, drinking diet soda leads to cravings for sweets and sugary snacks.

Another reason you're slugging diet soft drinks but not seeing the pounds come off? You feel you're "saving" calories by drinking a zero-calorie drink, so you "spend" them elsewhere — on a side of onion rings. If you believe that choosing diet soda alone will help you lose weight, you're going to be sorely mistaken.

> Soda contains no nutrients, although it is ultra-acidic, about the same pH as vinegar.

The Way to Lose Weight:

The bottom line is this: Diet soda drinkers aren't thinner, they're fatter. Sharon

P. Fowler's study concluded that people who drink 1 to 2 cans of diet soda per day have a 54.5 percent higher risk for obesity, and that number climbs to 57.1 percent for more than 2 cans each day.

It's not realistic to believe that drinking diet soda is enough of a weight-loss game plan. If you're eating at a fast-food restaurant, ordering a diet soda versus a full-sugar soda is virtually irrelevant. Don't fool yourself into eating fried chicken just because you're enjoying a zero-calorie soda. While diet soda is certainly preferable to full-sugar soda,

The bottom line is this: Diet soda drinkers aren't thinner, they're fatter.

it isn't a weight-loss solution in any way. While research has estimated that soft drinks make up between 5.5 and 7 percent of the calories in an American diet, it's what you're eating that is likely where you're getting too many empty calories, fats and carbs.

And as the aforementioned study suggests, giving up diet soda or cutting back drastically on your intake will help you eat fewer calories and better resist sweets. This can be difficult when soda products are sold everywhere you go, including in millions of convenient vending machines. Nearly every office, business and school has a vending machine that dispenses soda. Coca-Cola and its bottling partners alone have about 10 million vending machines and coolers around the world. So what is your plan for drinking fewer diet sodas and thus, eating fewer calories afterward? Decide that you are going to have water with most meals when you would normally have soda. If you love the fizzy taste of a soda, drink sparkling water or club soda for a refreshing change with zero calories. If you are near your target weight or simply can't live without some soda, treat yourself just once a week — not once a day. And when you buy cases of soda at the store, look for the new mini cans that come in 7.5- to 8-ounce sizes.

Truly, most dieters who give up soft drinks all together say they don't even miss them. And although the jury is still out on the damaging health effects of diet soda's artificial sweeteners, many health experts strongly believe that these chemical sugars can increase the risk of cancer, brain tumors, multiple sclerosis, migraines, depression and more. So help your waistline and your overall health by giving up or cutting back on your diet soda intake.

Taking the Stairs Won't Offset Your Morning Muffin

The Misconception:

Recently, one woman discussed what she does to be healthy, including taking the stairs whenever she can. However, this woman is also a fast-food lover who frequents the drive-thru and the freezer at 7-Eleven and often eats very late at night. So while taking the stairs is a nice policy to have, unless she works on the 20th floor of her office building, she's fooling herself by thinking taking the stairs is going to help her lose any weight.

"Take the stairs" or "park on the far end of the parking lot and walk" are two maxims you'll often hear from people trying to lose weight. Unfortunately, as is habit with many dieters stuck in a weight-loss rut, they believe doing these small things is enough to counter their poor eating choices.

Don't make the mistake of thinking taking three flights of stairs to your office means you can have a 400-calorie apple-cinnamon muffin for breakfast. A small effort does not equal a big reward. Even a sizeable effort — such as going for a 3-mile run — doesn't give you license to eat something unhealthy. The only way to lose weight is to save calories, after all.

The Way to Lose Weight:

Once again, the misstep here is rewarding yourself for a job well done when you haven't done, well, anything. Taking the stairs is always preferable to the elevator, of course, but it isn't enough to help you shed pounds. A better course of action is to start wearing a pedometer daily to measure how many steps you're taking and how many calories you're burning.

Pedometers usually clip to your belt or your pocket — any spot where they will be perpendicular to the ground. They come in a variety of styles and price points — for less than $20 you can get a sleek, simple device that counts steps and calculates calories burned. Deluxe models play music, feature audio, and allow you to upload your daily stats into your computer to track your progress and meet goals. Many new mP3 players come with built-in pedometers, as well. You'll want to reference consumer reports that test the efficiency and accuracy of different makes and models.

You'll quickly discover that climbing a few flights of stairs amounts to a handful of calories burned — certainly not enough to justify a fat-laden muffin. Wearing a pedometer might actually inspire you to start walking more, such as taking half your lunch break to go for a walk.

> Don't reward yourself for a job well done when you haven't done, well, anything.

Once you know how many calories you're burning, you can better map out your meals. Eating a quarter of a muffin might satisfy your sweet tooth, for instance. Better yet, try a bowl of oatmeal with a sprinkle of brown sugar or two whole wheat toaster waffles with a tablespoon of peanut butter, which will give you energy and brainpower for your day.

Don't Save Calories *Here*, Only to Spend Them *There*!

The Misconception:

You join a friend for dinner at your neighborhood bar and grill. You pass on the high-fat, high-calorie burgers, tacos and pasta dishes and settle on a healthier option: a salad. You even know better than to order the barbecue-ranch salad, with its unhealthy toppings and dressing. Since you're eating a low-calorie salad as your meal, you decide you can splurge on a frozen strawberry margarita.

You often make these same tradeoffs when it comes to your sweet tooth, as well. You decide that you can treat yourself to dessert if you have a low-calorie lunch.

And you wonder why you're not losing weight? Again, slimming down is simply a matter of burning more calories than you're taking in — which means you need to cut back, not just save calories in one area only to spend them in another! Not to mention that alcohol and sweets offer zero nutritional value. (And please don't try and say there's fruit juice in your margarita.)

Your major mistake is poor planning. Every meal requires a game plan, especially when you're dining out and healthy choices aren't always plentiful. If you're keeping a food diary (which is critical to weight loss), you should go into each breakfast, lunch or dinner knowing approximately how many calories you can "spend" on that meal to meet your total for the day. Spend them wisely, on food with nutritious value to it. If you're able to save a few hundred calories by ordering a filling low-calorie meal, do not shoot yourself in the foot by spending those calories on a sugary drink or dessert.

It's these tricky tradeoffs that keep you from getting to your desired weight.

The Way to Lose Weight:

Your goal is to cut calories wherever and whenever you can to get to a daily amount that allows you to lose weight and burn fat. Keeping track of how many calories are in what you eat and drink is the very best way to cut back and drop pounds. And once you know how much you need daily, you can also maintain your weight loss for a lifetime. Saving calories in one area to spend them in another is simply undermining your efforts.

For one, studies have shown again and again that people dramatically underestimate the number of calories in the foods they eat. Thus, you may think your "healthy" lunch has fewer calories than it really does, so when you indulge in the high-calorie margarita, you're actually taking in much more than you thought.

Every meal requires a game plan, especially when you're dining out and healthy choices aren't always plentiful.

Practice planning ahead for how many calories you'll spend on each meal. Consider any starters (soup or salad, perhaps), your main course, sides and beverages. For example, have water. Zero calories. Cross "beverages" off your list. Have a small side salad to start. Calories: 150. Have a 250-calorie turkey sandwich, hold the mayo, and you're at 400 calories. Now let's say you had budgeted 500 calories for this meal. You could spend that last 100 calories on a cookie, which provides a few moments of enjoyment, or you could save those last 100 calories. If you make this same choice every day, or every meal, you will see the difference on the scale and in the mirror at the end of the week — guaranteed.

The other reason you can't save calories to spend them on unhealthy foods on a daily basis is because there will be a few times a year when you actually need to employ this technique. Certain holidays and special occasions, such as a birthday, Thanksgiving or New Year's Eve, mean you will want to indulge in a rich dessert, buttery mashed potatoes or a few glasses of champagne. If you know you're going to spend a few hundred calories on these treats, you will need to plan throughout the day and week to cut back in other areas. Treating yourself, rarely and only when the occasion is meaningful, shows a healthy and well-balanced approach to eating. You're not using to food to celebrate, per se, but you're enjoying a special moment with loved ones that includes a dietary indulgence. This is OK on certain occasions, as long as you plan ahead.

Vitamins and Supplements Aren't Magic

The Misconception:

You eat from the drive-thru three days a week and spend more time on the couch than a teenager with a new video game, yet you take a complete multivitamin. Vitamins and supplements can help if you are deficient in certain areas, but too many Americans are under the false impression that a multivitamin or dietary supplement is a substitute for poor nutrition, lack of exercise or unhealthy lifestyle choices.

For example, a particular woman, who is a vegetarian, proudly showed off a freezer-size bag of vitamins she took. Are all those pills really necessary? "Well, I'm going to live longer," she remarked. However, this woman also smoked cigarettes, a pack a day at times, which puts her health at greater risk than could ever be compensated for with vitamins. In fact, smoking decreases the body's absorption of nutrients, such as calcium, vitamin C and magnesium, which are often deplete in vegetarians to begin with. This woman needed to wake up and realize she was negating any good that taking vitamins might do.

The reality is, if you smoke, drink in excess, don't get enough sleep, and forego a balanced diet, no multivitamin or supplement in the world is going to magically transform you. And no vitamin is going to help you lose weight if you're not getting a proper diet full of nutrients your body needs.

When you eat nutrient-rich food, like fresh fruits and veggies, high-protein lean meats, and fiber-filled beans, your body has to get to work burning fat and converting those nutrients into energy. When you eat processed and sugary foods that lack nutritional value, your body thinks, *What the heck is all this?* and stores fat cells instead.

The Way to Lose Weight:

Think of what you put into your body like the fuel you put in a car. If you had a beautiful new car you wanted to keep running at peak performance, you would use the best gas, oil, and other products. You wouldn't pour old, dirty oil into the car and expect it to run the way it was designed to. Your body is the same way.

First, if you're a smoker, get help to quit today. There's no sense in eating better if you're ingesting tar and nicotine.

To kickstart a sluggish metabolism, maintain your energy and inspire the body to burn fat cells, you must eat a balanced diet. The better you eat, the better your body works and the faster you'll lose weight. And you'll find that it only takes a few short weeks for your body to stop craving fatty and sugary processed foods. Some foods that pack meganutrients include low-fat yogurt, spinach, salmon, berries, avocados, whole grains, bell peppers, and olive oil.

Despite eating an array of fresh, low-fat foods, you may still be deficient in certain areas. According to the Dietary Guidelines for Americans, adults are most often deficient in calcium, magnesium, and vitamins A, C, and E. It is tough for most people to get their daily totals of vitamin E, for example, from food alone, so adding a multivitamin may be beneficial. Some nutrients and minerals, like vitamin A, however, are detrimental if you overdo them, so always check with your doctor before taking a supplement.

There are no quick fixes or magic vitamins to substitute for a healthy diet. Get real about the changes to your habits you must make to lose weight and use vitamins to fill in small gaps here and there as recommended by your doctor.

Going Cold Turkey Can Cause Cravings

The Misconception:

You crave salty chips, ice cream, chocolate, or bread. You recognize that you'll never lose weight by indulging your every craving, so you cut these foods out of your diet. No more sweets, chips, or starchy carbs. You're going cold turkey. The only problem is the cravings don't subside immediately and after a few days you feel like you'll freak out if you don't have a piece of chocolate or a buttery croissant. When your craving gets the best of you, you don't have one small bite of chocolate, you eat the entire bar, plus some chocolate-chip cookies. An inkling for sweets turns into a full-blown binge, and you've not only blown your calorie count for the day but you feel like a complete failure.

For most people, going cold turkey with food isn't realistic. Just like quitting smoking or drinking, eliminating the unhealthy foods you crave most is going to be a process and you may not succeed on the first try. For one, your body may be addicted to them. When you eat high-fat or sugary foods, your brain releases dopamine and other pleasure chemicals that make you feel good. When you deprive yourself of these foods, your body shifts into hedonism mode, demanding what makes it feel good.

And second, people have a tendency to want what they can't have, what is "forbidden." When you go cold turkey from your favorite foods, you dwell on thoughts of those more, until you give in to your craving and seriously overeat.

> People report having two to four craving episodes per week, and roughly 80 to 85 percent of these episodes lead to eating the desired food.

You're not alone in this behavior by any means. Food cravings — defined as "an intense desire to consume a particular food that is difficult to resist" — reportedly occur in 58 to 97 percent of the population, according to a study in the journal *Obesity*. The same report claims that individuals who experience food cravings report having two to four craving episodes per week, and roughly 80 to 85 percent of these episodes lead to eating the desired food.

Clearly, cravings are a very common occurrence, so it's simply not realistic to think you're going to eliminate your most-craved foods all together. And with the body's reinforcing response to eating bad foods, it's not a matter of willpower so much as it is science.

> **You don't have to be Superman or Jennifer Aniston when it comes to willpower, you just have to be smarter than your cravings.**

The good news is cravings do retreat over time. The above study from the journal *Obesity* found that its subjects' cravings decreased after the fifth or sixth week of being on a restricted diet.

The key is to develop balanced eating habits you can live with, instead of totally depriving yourself of certain items. You need to create a new lifestyle, instead of imaging that you'll never eat another ice cream sandwich again.

The Way to Lose Weight:

Some research studies have suggested that denying yourself certain foods makes the cravings for those exact foods worse. That's why a small treat can quickly result in a binge. And when you fall off the diet wagon with a great big thud, it really saps your motivation to get back on. For the majority of people, it's unrealistic to maintain that you're quitting sweets or carbs completely. You don't want to create the "forbidden fruit" mentality that makes the off-limits items seem even more desirable to you.

First, never restrict your diet to the point that you're ravenous. This is one of the most common mistakes dieters make, and it leads to overeating and goals that are unattainable. The idea isn't to crash diet by eating 1,200 calories a day, it's to evolve your eating habits to a level you can maintain as a lifestyle. Set a target amount of calories for each day and aim to stay right around that number. Surround yourself with healthy snacks to satisfy your hunger and stave off feelings of starvation.

Then, don't deprive yourself of the foods you love, just eat them in small quantities. A magazine interview with Jennifer Aniston once discussed how she opened a bag of Doritos from the mini bar in her hotel and ate one single chip. One. Now that takes some serious self-control. Most anyone else would have eaten the whole bag. But you don't have to be Superman or Jennifer Aniston when it comes to willpower, you just have to be smarter than your cravings. Eat pre-portioned amounts of the treats you crave, such as the 100-calorie packs of cookies, crackers and chips sold at all grocery stores. Everything from Reese's Peanut Butter Cups to Pringles now come in 100-calorie snack sizes. Allow yourself *just one* of these packages when the craving for something sweet or salty feels truly overwhelming.

Or, find healthy versions of what you crave. If you're an ice cream addict, try low-calorie, low-fat ice cream sandwiches from brands like Skinny Cow. Some dieters find that their sweet tooth can be satisfied by eating fruit instead of sugar. Try putting pineapple slices or halved peaches on the grill for a warm, sweet treat without high fructose corn syrup.

Better yet, treat yourself with something other than food. When you reach a certain numbers of milestone days without giving in to a craving, celebrate. A new item of clothing, a manicure and pedicure, or tickets to a concert or sporting event are all examples. Make a tradeoff that's actually healthy — give up fatty, sugary treats in favor of a non-food indulgence that causes happiness and relaxation instead of guilt!

Are You a Snacking Chef?

The Misconception:

Because frequent dining out throws a wrench in weight loss for many dieters, you make meals for yourself to help cut calories and fat. When you make sauces and meals at home you can regulate how much, if any, cream, butter, dressing and mayonnaise go into your food. You might make slow-cooker chili, grilled chicken tacos, or pasta with homemade sauce. Now that you've cut way back on eating out, fast-food and happy hour bar food you'd expect the pounds to start falling off, right? So why aren't they?

There is a reason so many well-known chefs — Gordon Ramsey, Jamie Oliver, Rachel Ray and many others — have publicly struggled with their weight. You might wonder, how can top chefs be overweight and obese while running around a hot kitchen all day? The reality is, cooking, for chefs of any caliber, means talking and thinking about food all day, in addition to preparing, seasoning and tasting each dish. Also, you mindlessly snack while waiting for meat to brown or water to boil. Or maybe you sip on wine while cooking. All these factors lead to hundreds of extra calories. In fact, you may not even be hungry by the time your meal is ready, although you're going to eat it anyway!

Start *paying attention* when you cook. Are you constantly "taste testing" your chili every few minutes? Do you snack on shredded cheese while you're dicing taco toppings? Does licking the spatula after making a dessert date back to a childhood habit?

You're not Mario Batali, so you don't need to be tasting your food every two minutes to make sure it's seasoned "just right."

What's the point in preparing a healthy meal for yourself or your family if you're snacking the whole time, adding hundreds of extra calories? And I'd be willing to bet those calories and grams of fat and carbs are going largely forgotten when you take a mental or written tally of what you ate that day. Wake up! Snacking while cooking is sabotaging your weight loss and going too easily overlooked.

The Way to Lose Weight:

Once again, it's time to start being accountable for your bad diet habits. Hello, you're not Mario Batali (and you wouldn't want to weigh as much as the Croc-wearing celebrity chef, anyhow), so you don't need to be tasting your food every two minutes to make sure it's seasoned "just right." Take a bite or two as necessary, then defer to your spouse, significant other or kids to tell you whether something needs more salt or more spice.

> Just like the old adage, "Don't grocery shop while you're hungry," don't cook while you're starving either. Start cooking before you're hungry.

Just like the old adage, "Don't grocery shop while you're hungry," don't cook while you're starving either. Start making a meal before you're hungry so the food is ready by the time you're eager to eat. If it's too late and you're already hungry, set aside a small plate of veggies, such as carrots or crunchy cucumber slices, to enjoy while you cook. A spoonful of peanut butter or a few crackers can also hold you over for a while so you aren't tempted to lick the bowl after making banana bread.

Another dieters' trick is chewing a piece of peppermint gum while cooking. Some studies have shown that mint flavor and smell may suppress appetite for a short period of time. The majority of what your brain perceives as taste is actually smell, so the idea is that if you saturate your sense of smell with a strong odor, like mint, the smell of food will be less appealing, and you're less likely to eat more than you need. In one study from Wheeling Jesuit University, 40 people sniffed peppermint every two hours for five days, then sniffed a placebo for the next five days. During the week they smelled the peppermint, they consumed 1,800 fewer calories. And even if peppermint doesn't distract your appetite, having a piece of gum in your mouth will stop you from putting other food there.

Finally, don't let wine or other alcohol contribute hundreds of needless calories while you cook, especially because alcohol whets the appetite. Save the wine for the meal (and limit yourself to just one glass), and have a Perrier or glass of water nearby to keep your hands and mouth busy.

Emotio

al Eating

Chapter 3 · Emotional Eating

Ever heard of eating your feelings? Emotional eating is a huge problem in most diets gone awry, because the very nature of being overweight causes stress, anxiety, sadness and loneliness, which all contribute to the cycle of emotional eating.

Anything from relationship problems to unemployment to depression to work-related stress can lead to emotional eating. And, unfortunately, emotional eaters are typically only interested in fatty or sugary snacks that completely derail their diet plans.

As this chapter reveals, *positive* emotions and people you love may be causing you to emotionally eat as well. You'll learn to recognize the triggers that lead you to overeat out of celebration, or the friends and loved ones who mean well but are actually wreaking havoc on your weight.

This chapter reveals fascinating facts about how eating in a social setting, with your significant other or family members, or around coworkers can determine how much and what you eat. You'll also learn about how your gender affects your calorie intake, as well as your attitudes toward food.

In reality, emotional eating revolves around having a very unhealthy relationship with food — using it as a coping mechanism, a comfort, a distraction from your problems, a means to fit in, or a reward. Whether you're overeating in a group of friends or pigging out on late-night junk food when you're home alone, you'll finally be confronted with your bad habits and given a variety of ways to make better food and lifestyle choices.

Because emotional eating habits are some of the most difficult to change (they often date back decades, to childhood), these are also the behaviors that frustrate people and keep them from losing significant weight. Feeling powerless to food and your weight is a daily struggle. But learning the emotional triggers, people and situations that lead you to make unhealthy choices is the only way to break the nasty cycle of overeating that causes sadness and anxiety and, in turn, more overeating.

Wouldn't you love to feel in control of your eating habits for *once* in your life? Wouldn't you love to find other, healthy ways to address stress, conflict, personal issues or to celebrate, without ruining your weight-loss efforts? Read on to figure out how to eat for nutrition and not to feed your feelings.

Instant Diet Makeover Tips:

▸ Try not to eat while watching television, driving, reading or any other activity. It can make you lose track of how much you're eating.

▸ Schedule an event that you would like to lose weight for, such as your birthday, a vacation, or high school reunion. This gives you a set date to work toward.

▸ Instead of fixating on all the "bad stuff," write down all the physical qualities you like about yourself and the good things you have done for your body.

▸ Ginger, cinnamon, nutmeg, and vanilla are all good additions to food in order to curb a sweet tooth.

▸ Adopt a relaxation technique, such as yoga or deep breathing, to reduce your stress levels and lose weight.

▸ Don't be too hard on yourself if you stumble along the way. Just remember that tomorrow is another day, and you can get back on track.

▸ Write this down! The gratification of gradual weight loss will be much more satisfying than the instant gratification of food.

Emotional Eating Makes You Feel *Worse*

The Misconception:

You got fired, you got a promotion, you broke up with your boyfriend, your team won the Super Bowl — so you eat half a pizza. You tell yourself, "I *deserve* this." You use food to both celebrate and to help you lick your wounds. What the heck kind of sense does that make?

Yet many overweight and obese people admit that one of their greatest diet pitfalls is using unhealthy food as a coping or reward mechanism. Recognize where this behavior originates from. Might it date back to your childhood, when your mom would cook your favorite fried chicken after you did well on a test, or soothe you with a bowl of ice cream when you were sad?

Crying into a glass of wine and a pint of ice cream after a breakup might make you feel better initially, but you'll loathe yourself in the morning. Eating for comfort after a bad day or a misfortune only compounds feelings of letdown or negativity and creates new stress in an already stressful situation.

And why would you want the glow of new job to be outshined by the guilt you feel for eating a pound of Buffalo wings at your celebratory happy hour?

The notion that you are deserving of a mega-calorie meal because of circumstances largely out of your control is preventing you from losing the weight that brings you down. How many times have you heard: "I eat because I'm sad, and then I'm sad because I'm fat"?

> Food is *not* your friend. A burrito doesn't help you celebrate, and it doesn't make for a very good shoulder to cry on either.

The fact of the matter is, when you use food as a reward or as a comfort you give calories the power to control you every time something goes right or wrong. Now that's pretty sad.

Also, constantly treating yourself to high-calorie foods can lead to overeating as a lifestyle. A ground-breaking report from the 2009 meeting for the Society for Neuroscience showed that rats that were fed a high-calorie diet of items like bacon, sausage and cheesecake had diminished response in the pleasure centers of their brains over time. As the animals' brain reward circuits became less responsive, they continued to overeat and become more and more obese. Their brains actually began to mimic those of rats addicted to drugs as they became addicted to high-calorie foods. Thus, letting emotional eating become a habit will continue to contribute to being overweight. You must get real about breaking this cycle!

The Way to Lose Weight:

Like every little white diet lie we tell ourselves, becoming conscious of our bad habits and triggers is the best step toward losing weight. The next time you're casually looking through the fridge, ask yourself, "Am I really hungry?" If you just ate an hour or two ago, think about whether something else is going on in your life that might be causing emotional hunger.

Remind yourself that food is *not* your friend. A burrito doesn't help you celebrate, and it doesn't make for a very good shoulder to cry on either. Be honest with yourself about these negative coping patterns, and look for healthy ways of rewarding yourself or dealing with stress or sadness.

Had a great day? Go shopping and treat yourself to a new pair of shoes. Do something that makes you feel great, other than overindulging in food, like getting a massage. Meet a friend for a drink — one drink — and soak in the congratulations.

Ask yourself, "Am I really hungry?" If you just ate an hour or two ago, think about whether something else might be causing emotional hunger.

Had a crappy day? Sweat it out at the gym or go for a run. Exercise is the number one stress reliever. And obviously, when you're exercising you're doing something beneficial for your body, as opposed to indulging in a calorie-packed meal.

Or, try warming up with a hot bath, soak in the Jacuzzi, warm blanket and a book, bowl of soup, or hot tea. Warmth, especially liquids, is proven to help calm and relax people. Tea is a favorite natural tool for determining if you're eating out of emotions or hunger. If you think you're feeling hungry, try drinking a mug of hot tea, such as chamomile. If within a few minutes you begin to feel relaxed and your hunger pangs subside, you'll know that emotions were trying to trick you into eating when you weren't really hungry.

Also, remind yourself that food does not provide emotional support, loved ones do. If you're going through an emotional or difficult time, call a friend and have a good cry. Better still, combine calorie-burning physical activity with emotional support and go for a walk together. Many emotional eaters equate food with love, so the love and support of a real person helps put an end to that. Just getting a hug from a friend can keep you away from the chips and cookies.

Finally, head off emotional eating at the pass. Figure out which types of emotions and circumstances lead you to eat out of emotion, rather than hunger. The five most typical emotions or states that cause overeating are loneliness, boredom, anger, stress, and fatigue. If your hand ends up in the bottom of the Snackwells after a fight with your sister, make a mental note of it. Then you will be able to anticipate and stop emotional eating down the road.

Work Food is Getting in the Way of Weight Loss

The workplace is one spot where there always seems to be a reason for food. A coworker's birthday merits cake and ice cream; a promotion calls for happy hour; the holidays mean homemade fudge in the breakroom; Monday morning meetings incorporate bagels and cream cheese. Team-building and bonding often include group lunches, potlucks, or company picnics. The misconception is that in order to interact and connect with your coworkers, you must indulge in unhealthy food and large portions. Wrong. This attitude is keeping you from a doable diet!

What's the point of exercising and eating right — having a salad or a healthy sandwich for lunch several days a week — only to be thwarted when Sheri from accounting brings in freshly baked cookies? Get rid of the notion that you are showing loyalty and camaraderie to Sheri and your other coworkers by eating cookies.

Also, as odd as it may sound, many people are afraid to be

seen as "the healthy one" in a group. If you are concerned that coworkers will roll their eyes when everyone is ordering cheeseburgers and you ask for salmon, you have to remember that getting to your healthy weight requires daily choices that only you can make. Eating right is not always easy — or popular! — but you will be happier, healthier, more active, and live longer. Your coworkers wish they had your resolve and healthy attitude.

> Get rid of the notion that you are showing loyalty and camaraderie to your coworkers by eating junk food.

The Way to Lose Weight:

You can bond with your officemates and still stick to your diet plan, you just need to exercise a little willpower. When Sheri comes around with a plate of her homemade chocolate chip cookies and offers you one, politely decline, but with a compliment: "Oh, no thank you, but they look wonderful. You are such a good baker!"

Now, there are some well-meaning people who won't take no for an answer. If Sheri presses you further and you don't feel comfortable turning her down, take the cookie, but immediately throw it away when she is gone. Don't feel guilty! You should never eat something you know will undermine your weight loss simply to preserve someone else's feelings.

The same goes for workplace celebrations or meetings. Stick to your guns. Ask for a small sliver of birthday cake and eat only a few bites. You don't have to skip the office happy hour — just sip on one light beer or seltzer water with a squeeze of lemon. If you're having a hard time passing up the mozzarella cheese sticks, order a small side salad to have something to snack on. If the office hosts a potluck, offer to bring a tasty, healthy dish like veggie chili or a Mediterranean salad, so you'll have something to enjoy in case no one else makes anything healthy. And, if your client meeting includes a spread of muffins, bagels and fruit, load up on the fruit. Don't indulge in a 400-calorie muffin just because everyone else at the conference table is.

Remind yourself that what you eat does not make you part of the team — your friendly personality, attitude, and work performance do.

Let People See
You Eat — Healthy

The Misconception:

You attend a romantic date, birthday dinner with friends, charity event, or group lunch with coworkers. When the menus are passed around, you begin to feel anxious that you'll order a hamburger when everyone else is ordering a salad or you'll look like a pig for eating everything that is served. You're so worried about what others are thinking while you eat that you order only a small side salad or whatever everyone at the table orders, only to overeat or binge on junk food later when you're alone. When you finally get to eat in the privacy of your own home, you feel relieved and comforted by the food.

This type of emotional eating is triggered by anxiety and is most prevalent in women, who often worry about being judged for eating or not appearing "ladylike" to others. "When I eat in a group, I am convinced that everyone is thinking, 'Why is she eating so much? She doesn't need to eat that,'" said one woman who admits to this behavior.

Another woman explained that she enjoys looking "disciplined" when she meets her college sorority sisters for dinner once a month, so she orders something very small, like a side of cottage cheese, but then pigs out on Snickers and Coca-Cola when she gets home. She found herself steadily gaining weight, although she maintained the outward appearance of being on a restricted diet.

And who hasn't experienced this: Not ordering what you really want on a date because you're afraid to look gluttonous in front of a stranger you're trying to impress. Unfortunately, not eating doesn't make you look refined; it's only a false reality, and an unhealthy one if you're snacking when you get home.

Anxiety about eating in front of others, only to pig out later, is not only keeping you from losing weight, it's actually an indication of disordered eating. The relief you feel when you overeat alone later is a sign that eating is becoming an obsession. You cannot let food control you! While it is important to exert self-control when you are eating in a group, don't let others' opinions or what they are eating affect you. Stick to your diet plan, don't give in to food peer pressure, and enjoy your meal. Your company won't be assessing what or how much you ate or didn't eat — they will appreciate that you have a healthy relationship with food.

The Way to Lose Weight:

Look around you the next time you go out to eat with friends, family or coworkers. Everyone is eating. This is because food is a necessary and normal part of everyday life; however, you can't allow it to control you.

Try not to inquire or pay attention to what other people are ordering. Someone who is taking a constant poll of the table can be very annoying. If you are worried that the prime rib is too much of a diet splurge but a salad sounds too meager to fill you up, try something in the middle, such as a fish fillet with a vegetable or soup on the side. And trust that no one is going to remember what you order, either way.

> Not eating doesn't make you look refined; it's only a false reality, and an unhealthy one if you're snacking when you get home.

When you attend a group dinner with a set menu of several courses, tell yourself you will eat a little of each course so you don't overdo it but still feel satiated. The convenient thing about a multi-course meal is that the courses are timed out so your body has a chance to feel full. At a multi-course catered meal, skip the basket of dinner rolls and butter. Salad dressings are generally served from a boat, so you are able to pour yourself only a small amount. When dessert comes, have a bite or two, then flag down a waiter to remove your plates as soon as you are satisfied.

If you are concerned about appearing refined or ladylike on a date or in a group, consider that being polite isn't about what you eat or how much, it's about how you eat. Order what you want, but chew and eat your food slowly. Shoveling dinner into your mouth isn't attractive, even if dinner is a salad. If you're worried about appearing sloppy, avoid messy meals that require eating with your hands, such as ribs or crab legs. Having good manners and eating at a reasonable pace will make you less self-conscious and able to enjoy eating in a group.

> Don't let others' opinions or what they are eating affect you. Stick to your diet plan, don't give in to food peer pressure, and enjoy your meal.

Still, it is not totally out of the question that an ungraceful dinner companion would comment on what you are eating or how much. Let's say after you order someone asks, "I thought you were on a diet?" Don't take offense. This person is simply projecting his or her own insecurities about food and weight onto you. Your weight-loss journey starts with being in control of your diet, health and nutrition and never being a slave to bad food habits. Try responding with something like, "You know, I am just working on having a healthy relationship with food."

And practice what you preach! Never comment on or chuckle at what another diner orders — even when you start noticing your friends and family making the diet mistakes you're reading about in these pages! When your friend orders a salad with a side of onion rings, keep your comments to yourself. (You can always give him or her a copy of this book later.)

Your friends and loved ones will appreciate the kind of relationship you are striving to have with food — one of balance, never starvation or deprivation, and of honesty.

Is a Friend or Loved One Sabotaging Your Weight Loss?

The Misconception:

You're ready to put an end to your bad diet habits and start losing weight, so naturally your friends and family will be there to support you, right? So why do you feel pressured to eat more than you want at every family get-together, or why does your husband roll his eyes and say, "Oh, she doesn't eat *real* food anymore" when you pass on the appetizer at dinner with friends? When you don't give in, you feel ridiculed and put down, and when you do indulge, you feel guilty and resentful toward your loved ones.

While it is natural to expect that the ones who care for you would want to help you in your efforts to lose weight, many people find that certain friends and family members actually sabotage their weight loss — intentionally and unintentionally. Take a look at the person in question — typically, he or she is also struggling with weight, overeating and a sedentary lifestyle. Some people feel better about their unhealthy lifestyle choices when you live the same way. After all, no one wants to be the only one at the table who orders dessert or grabs a third slice of pizza.

If the person undercutting your efforts is your spouse or close friend, jealousy and insecurity are probably involved. If you begin to lose a lot of weight, people will compliment and praise you, and your husband, wife, or best friend will feel left out, overlooked, and it may reinforce his or her own insecurities. Many times, the person you are closest to has long been your partner in crime when it comes to unhealthy eating. He or she will feel isolated and jealous when you start making better food choices and pass on the beer-and-pizza-Saturdays that have become your tradition. Your spouse, for one, may not want you to lose weight, because he or she is afraid that you will become more desirable to other people or be tempted to cheat.

When it comes to family members sabotaging your weight loss, culture and tradition may also come into play. In Greek, Latino and Italian families, for instance, being together and enjoying each other's company often means huge spreads of food. Overindulging is thought of as a sign of health and happiness (when quite the opposite is true). It can be uncomfortable if your relatives are constantly pushing food at you or commenting how you're so thin "you might blow away" when you are actually trying to lose weight. Try not to take it personally; they mean well, many people simply equate a big meal with love and a family bonding experience.

The odd thing about our culture is that while it would be considered wildly inappropriate and cruel to make fun of an overweight person diving into a plate of nachos, it is acceptable to poke fun at the person on a diet who declines the nachos. A friend might find it perfectly fine to mock you, saying, "Oh, you eat like a bird," or, "C'mon, one bite of nachos won't hurt you." This friend may be well-meaning, albeit inconsiderate, or he or she may be jealous of your self-control and weight-loss progress. Whatever the case, don't let friends and loved ones undermine your strength and will. And don't give in just for the sake of fitting in. This is your body and your health, not anyone else's.

The Way to Lose Weight:

Whether the person sabotaging your weight loss is well-meaning and oblivious or truly conniving, you must have a frank talk with him or her. Avoid making the person feel guilty or like his or her lifestyle is inferior to your new, healthy one. Emphasize that you are making these changes for you, to be healthier, happier and live longer.

Explain that you are committed to breaking out of bad

habits, losing weight and keeping it off, which is going to require a complete lifestyle makeover. This means that some things will change. You will be ordering and cooking different types of food now. You will be passing on the bread basket. You may not be joining your buddies for margaritas and Mexican food like you used to. You may pass on Sunday brunch in favor of a hike or workout session. Your friend or loved one has two choices: to accept your new lifestyle or participate in it. Losing weight and getting active are always easier with a partner, so invite your spouse or friend to join you in your weight-loss efforts.

> Remind your loved ones that you will be the same person, only happier, after you lose weight. You will need their support throughout this process.

That person may feel intimidated, and if your offer is declined, reinforce that you will still need his or her full support. If your spouse does the cooking or grocery shopping, he or she needs to respect your mission by keeping fatty, sugary foods out of the house and making an effort to cook smaller portions of healthier food. Take initiative by compiling some nutritional recipes you would like your spouse to try.

If your spouse or friend doesn't want to give up fast-food, you can set a good example by ordering a salad or grilled chicken sandwich the next time you go through the drive-thru. Don't give in to unhealthy foods, even if this person tries to persuade you that one little burger won't kill you. Stay strong! People who have successfully lost weight repeatedly say that the happiness they get from being healthy and thin far outweighs the short-lived enjoyment they got from eating bad foods. Plus, healthy eating often catches on, so be the one in your family or social group who starts the smart-eating trend.

Losing weight can be intimidating for others. Friends and significant others may fear that once you lose weight you'll be distracted by attention from new people or that you'll have nothing in common any longer. They simply need reassurance. Remind your loved ones that you will be the same person, only happier, after you lose weight. You will need their support throughout this process. Once loved ones are onboard with your lifestyle adjustments, they can help you stay accountable by checking in with you and reminding you of your goals when temptation arises.

Fend Off the Late-Night Snack Attack

The Misconception:

You try to eat a healthy diet throughout the day, including dinner in the early evening. But after a few hours of relaxing at home, you're hungry again, just a short time before you're due to go to sleep. So you sometimes have a late-night snack. You're a weekday late-night snacker, and you feel justified in eating something while relaxing in front of the TV after a long day at work or with your family.

Or, you might be a weekend late-night snacker. On weekend evenings you're staying up later, perhaps going out with friends until the early morning hours. Naturally, if you eat dinner at 7 p.m., you'll be hungry again at 2 a.m. So what's the problem?

The myth is that it's so much worse to eat late at night; however, it's not as much *when* you eat but *what* you're eating. The real issue with late-night snacking is that the only places that are open at that time are the fast-food drive-thru, 24-hour Mexican food, and convenience stores. And who ever grabbed a piece of fruit when they had an urge for a late-night snack while watching TV at home? More than likely, you're going to be reaching for a crunchy, cheesy, starchy snack late in the evening. Think about it: What was the last thing you ate late-night? A burrito, a bag of chips, a fast-food burger, a Denny's Grand Slam Breakfast? Have you ever ordered or made yourself a salad at 2 a.m.? Didn't think so.

Another problem with late-night eating is the alcohol factor. Many times, a late night out involves drinking with friends, which boosts the appetite for unhealthy food and seriously suppresses our normal willpower. You might never eat half a pizza for lunch, but late at night, after a few beers, nothing sounds better. Midnight munchies also lead to health problems and disrupted sleep for many people. Eating and lying down shortly thereafter can worsen heartburn or acid reflux in people who are prone to these issues.

Late-night snacking is like eating an entire other meal for most people. Taco Bell has even made an advertising campaign around it, calling it "Fourth Meal"! Why watch what you eat so closely all day, only to sabotage yourself with a late-night taco combo? You'll wake up feeling guilty, knowing that you'll never lose the weight you want.

The Way to Lose Weight:

Interestingly, many dieticians and nutritionists say that late-night eating is their clients' biggest problem that keeps them from losing weight. They eat smart all day only to fall victim to midnight munchies. Does this sound like you?

Learn to ward of the late-night snack attack by determining why you're tempted to eat so late. There is an off-chance that you've restricted your calories so much throughout the day, and so you're actually hungry before bed. If so, try adding more fiber or protein to your dinner to feel fuller longer.

> It's not as much *when* you eat but *what* you're eating. Have you ever made yourself a salad at 2 a.m.? Didn't think so.

However, most late-night snackers are simply just emotional eaters. Loneliness, boredom and stress are three of the most typical emotions that cause eating for reasons other than hunger. When you're at home, late-night eating is commonly caused by boredom or the release of stress. Mindless, needless eating is generally accompanied by sitting on the couch with a movie, magazine or TV show. Also, weekday late-night eaters often enjoy the peace and quiet of eating their favorite snack foods alone, after their roommate, spouse or children have gone to sleep. After a stressful day, late-night snackers feel relaxed and comforted by a bowl of ice cream or bag of chips. Or, if you feel lonely late at night, you're turning to food as comfort.

> Find an activity that includes both hands so you won't have one hand on your book and the other in a bag of Doritos.

Weekend late-night eaters are dealing with the other side of emotional eating — eating in a social setting. Many dieters report late-night slices of pizza or drive-thru burgers after a night out with friends. And, as mentioned above, any alcohol you may have had during the night will increase your appetite.

The best way to stop emotional eating is to recognize it, anticipate it and head it off at the pass. To avoid eating out of the desire for comfort, look for other things that fulfill this need, such as a bath or exchanging massages with your spouse. If you know you're going to be relaxing at home, find something to do with your hands other than eating, such as drinking a mug of tea. Warm liquids are also said to have a calming and de-stressing effect that helps you unwind and get ready for a good night of sleep. Or, find an activity that includes both hands so you won't have one hand on your book and the other in a bag of Doritos. Type an email to a friend or knit. Cleaning can also be a good stress reliever that keeps you busy and out of the fridge. Getting up off the couch and going for a walk is also a good distraction. After 10 minutes, the craving for a snack should have passed.

When you're heading out with friends on the weekends, you need to devise a strategy to avoid late-night eating ahead of time. If your friends typically hit up the Jack-in-the-Box drive-thru or 24-hour pizza joint at midnight, excuse yourself and head home before they go. You will find it difficult to be the only person not eating if you stay. If you distance yourself from the situation, the temptation to eat will be gone.

If your late-night craving is out of habit or boredom, remind yourself that it will pass and simply go to bed. Brushing your teeth can also stop you from eating anything else.

However, if you're still up after midnight, having not eaten since the early evening, you may have gone 6 or 7 hours without food. It is normal to feel hungry at that point. If your stomach is grumbling late at night and you're feeling like you're ready for a whole other meal, maybe it's time to go to bed a bit earlier.

Are You Eating Out and Pigging Out?

The Misconception:

One of your favorite things to do with friends is go out for dinner. You love to catch up, have a good conversation, and eat a delicious meal. You might split an appetizer, dessert or both. And because you're enjoying a night with friends, the incentive to linger after the meal is high, thus you usually have a few after-dinner drinks or a cappuccino, as well.

You want to maintain willpower but you feel like the relaxed, social atmosphere makes it difficult to refuse a dessert or drink. You're afraid your friends will think you're not fun if you turn down food or alcohol. You leave feeling great about spending time with friends but wonder if these events are sabotaging your diet.

The issue is that many social events revolve around eating — and you are eating to please others. To compound this problem, restaurant portions in the U.S. have nearly tripled in size over the last few decades. Have you ever heard someone who traveled abroad complain about the small portion sizes in Europe? That's because in Italy, for example, meat, pasta and vegetables are ordered and served as individual courses, whereas Americans are used to having all three piled high in the same dish. In the U.S., you're eating far more at a restaurant than you would if you were cooking for yourself at home. A recent study showed that people consume 50 percent more calories, fat and sodium when they eat out.

Also, consider who your dinner companions are, especially if you are female. A 2009 study in the journal *Appetite* studied the effects of eating in social settings on both men and women and discovered that women who ate in all-female groups ate significantly more than if they ate alone, on a date, or in a group that included men. When men were at the table, the women ate about 450 calories each. By contrast, in an all-female group, the number rose to about 750 calories. Interestingly, while men were not affected by the gender of their company, they consumed more than 700 calories per meal regardless, which was higher than all the women in the study.

The bottom line is social environments lead to poor impulse control and overeating. Surely you've heard the phrase "Eat, drink and be merry." If your mindset is that eating out with friends is an "indulgence" or treat, you're more likely to indulge in high-calorie food, desserts and drinks.

And social settings create peer pressure, even among friends. People who feel the need to eat to please others will always eat more in social situations.

> If your mindset is that eating out with friends is an "indulgence," you're more likely to indulge in high-calorie food, desserts and drinks.

The Way to Lose Weight:

Don't let something fun and positive — a night out with friends — turn into something bad that sabotages your weight-loss efforts. Being social and spending time with friends is good for your health, happiness and stress management, so you should never feel you have to pass on a dinner invitation just to lose weight. You just need to plan ahead, recognize the pitfalls of social gatherings, and be prepared to exercise some serious willpower.

One big mistake people make is barely eating all day in anticipation of dinner with friends. Then they're starving and they overeat. Instead, eat normally throughout the day and have a small snack before you leave for your dinner. According to Purdue University research, eating a pre-meal snack of a handful of peanuts about an hour before dinner will lead you to eat less total calories and fat during your main meal. Also, a broth-based soup or small side salad are good pre-meal choices.

To eat less, anticipate what you're going to order, so your eyes don't get bigger than your stomach when you're sitting at the table with all your friends. Most restaurant menus are online now, so check ahead of time and decide what you're going to have. Consider ordering an appetizer, such as steamed mussels or a Caprese salad, as your meal.

> Organizing a group meal in your home means consuming hundreds of calories less than if you were heading out to a restaurant.

And stay strong! Clearly, female impulse control is greatly affected when eating with other women. Be cautious that girls' night out doesn't turn into a 2,000-calorie food fest. And if you're a man, don't sabotage your diet by eating a high-calorie dinner just to fit in.

Both sexes should feel confident enough to say "No thanks" when a dinner companion suggests splitting the fried calamari or cheesecake. Alcohol and coffee drinks also rack up major calories, so order hot tea if everyone is having after-dinner drinks. If someone questions you, just say you don't feel like drinking and leave it at that. Remind yourself that no one will remember who ate or didn't eat what an hour after the meal, so never feel pressured to overindulge.

One big mistake people make is barely eating all day in anticipation of dinner with friends. Then they're starving and they overeat.

Another way to enjoy food and the company of friends while eating healthy and smart is to host a dinner party where you cook a majority of the dishes and provide the beverages. Cooking at home means eating smaller portions than you would at a restaurant and you can control what goes into each dish. This is a big benefit when you consider that many restaurant meals are prepared with unhealthy oils, butter, and creamy sauces. Serve courses that include fruits, vegetables, lean meats and whole grains, such as recipes taken from Mediterranean cuisine. Serve natural sparkling water, like Perrier, with several choices of garnish to avoid the empty calories of alcohol. Guests can feel free to bring wine or beer, but you'll have an option for sticking to your weight-loss program. Organizing a group meal in your home means consuming hundreds of calories less than if you were heading out to a restaurant.

Finally, try social activities that don't include eating! Duh! Do something exercise-related, such as arranging for a group bike ride, hike or entering a 5k with friends. Organize a weekend get-together at the beach, complete with Frisbee or a sand volleyball game. Or plan a museum visit, afternoon at the dog park, or trip to a landmark in your city. You'll be getting out of the house, off the couch, and doing something active with buddies. There are a million ways to enjoy the company and reap the health benefits of good friends without having to open the button on your pants afterwards!

Chapter 4

What's
Doesn'
Equal

"In" Always Thin"

What's "In" Doesn't Always Equal "Thin"

Have you ever noticed how certain words always seem to pop up when people are talking about losing weight, especially quick and easy methods? A new "celebrity" diet or "all-natural" product that claims to make the extra weight drop right off? An "organic" juice that flushes out toxins and eliminates unwanted fat? Perhaps it's a "low-fat" version of your favorite cookies, or maybe you read about the latest study that says eating chocolate is actually healthy for you. Fantastic! Now you don't have to give up the sweet snacks you love!

Unfortunately, these are just some of the many trendy diet buzzwords that lead people to believe they can make a very small effort to get big weight-loss results.

According to Merriam-Webster's Dictionary, the definition of a buzzword is "an important-sounding technical word or phrase, often of little meaning and used chiefly to impress laymen." Retailers and marketers know that trends and buzzwords like "fresh," "heart healthy" and "fat-free" make a huge impression on consumers, most times without delivering any real health or weight-loss benefits. While the FDA and other organizations are cracking down on what products can and can't be labeled with these terms, it's still up to you to see through the hype.

Don't be fooled! While switching to organic produce or mixing protein bars into your diet are personal choices, they aren't enough to drive weight loss. Once you recognize these tricky buzzwords, you'll learn to spot fad diets, the products that offer empty promises, as well as the products that actually cause weight *gain*.

You'll also learn about the bad eating behaviors triggered by buzzwords and trends that will shock and amaze you. For instance, did you know that studies have shown that people actually eat *more* of a product labeled low-fat or fat-free than they would its full-fat counterpart? Wise up to dieting's many buzzwords and quit fooling yourself into believing in the quick fix.

Losing weight and keeping it off for good is a measured process that includes self-awareness, knowledge, and the strength to make real lifestyle changes. Just know the results will be worth it — and friends and family will soon be coming to you for your weight-loss and diet secrets!

Instant Diet Makeover Tips:

▸ Disassociate diets with restriction and deprivation. Look at diets as eating the right foods in the right amounts.

▸ If you are always on the go, traveling, or on vacation, pack healthy snacks like an apple, dried fruits, nuts, or whole wheat crackers.

▸ "Enriched" foods have nutrients added to them that were lost during food processing. "Fortified" foods have nutrients added that were not originally present.

▸ Fruits and vegetables have a high fiber and water content, which means they fill you up and keep you full longer. Just do not confuse water loss with fat loss when you get on the scale.

▸ Fat is an important nutrient. Just make sure the fat you consume is the healthy, unsaturated kind found in fish, nuts, and seeds.

▸ Schedule rewards into your program to congratulate yourself for every positive step you make. If you include a healthy treat in your weight-loss plan so you don't feel deprived, try to keep these foods between 200 and 250 calories.

Eating "Organic" Won't Help You Shed Pounds

The Misconception:

One afternoon, a woman came into a neighborhood pizzeria wanting to order a salad. She asked, "Is the lettuce organic? Are the vegetables all organic?" The young guy working the counter told her yes, although he probably didn't know "organic" from "oregano." Then, the woman said, "Great, I'll have that salad … with two sides of Ranch dressing."

The misconception? That organic food is healthier for you — so much so, in fact, that its health benefits will somehow outweigh the negative effects of the 30-plus grams of fat in two sides of Ranch dressing.

Another great example of this delusion are the new organic cigarettes on the market. Even cigarette companies are trying to capitalize on this buzzword! Can Americans really be this dense to believe that organic tobacco is better for them? The truth is organic cigarettes actually contain higher levels of nicotine and tar than conventional cigarettes.

Back to the organic salad drenched in Ranch. Pouring four or five tablespoons of Ranch or any other creamy dressing onto your salad completely negates the purpose of eating a salad. You're better off with a slice of pizza. A salad is not going to help you lose weight until you get picky about what goes on it.

> Don't fool yourself into thinking cooking with organic food makes up for eating highly caloric meals.

Second, there is no evidence that organic produce is in any way nutritionally superior to conventionally grown food. In 2009, the London School of Hygiene & Tropical Medicine published the most extensive systematic review of organic foods to date in *The American Journal of Clinical Nutrition*. The researchers found organically and conventionally produced foods to be comparable in their nutrient content.

Any minor differences are "unlikely to be of any public health relevance," said Alan Dangour, one of the authors of the report. He added, "Our review indicates that there is currently no evidence to support the selection of organically over conventionally produced foods on the basis of nutritional superiority."

So, while organic growing processes may benefit the environment, the term "organic" does not mean "healthier" and won't help you lose weight. Grass-fed beef still has all the fat and calories of any other steak. If your favorite organic yogurt brand is made with whole milk, as many are, you're eating 150 to 200 calories and tons of fat in a few spoonfuls. You can't eat fatty salad dressing or deep-fried vegetables just because the produce was grown organically. Don't fool yourself into thinking cooking with organic food makes up for eating highly caloric meals.

The Way to Lose Weight:

If you prefer to buy organic produce and your budget allows for it, by all means. The most worthwhile organic products are the ones where you consume the whole of the item, such as bell peppers, apples, and meat. Something like an orange or a banana where you're peeling and discarding the skin won't be affected by organic growing processes. A great idea is growing your own tomatoes, peppers, squash, long beans or other produce right on your porch or in your backyard. Having an edible garden is easier to maintain than you might think and makes incorporating fresh, pesticide-free produce into your meals so convenient. You're much more inclined to toss some cherry tomatoes in with your fish if they're just a few steps away.

Many people falsely believe that simply shopping in the organic grocery aisle means they are eating healthy. But organic eating is really just a preference. To lose weight you must be smart about how you prepare and season your food.

These days, everything comes in an organic version. Just remind yourself that organic red meat doesn't have any fewer calories and an organic pie is still a pie.

Never deep fry anything! What good are organic zucchini if they're battered and fried. Skip cheese sauce on your veggies and opt for a sprinkle of parmesan and drizzle of olive oil if you want. Eating your produce raw is always best.

The rule of thumb with salad dressings is, ask for them on the side and use them sparingly. And if you need to ask for two sides of dressing, you're overdoing it on the dressing, the size of your salad, or both. Plus, less dressing means a fresher, crunchier salad, without all the extra vinaigrette drenching the lettuce in the bottom of the bowl.

Skip the creamy, fatty, mayo-based dressings and opt for a light vinaigrette instead. The monounsaturated fats in olive oil can help reduce the risk of heart disease — just use a light hand with oil-based dressings, once again. Still a better choice? Squeeze the juice of a fresh lemon over your salad greens for lots of flavor without calories or fat.

These days, everything comes in an organic version of the original, from red meat to milk to desserts. Just remind yourself that organic red meat doesn't have any fewer calories and an organic pie is still a pie, comprised of mostly butter and sugar. Include a few pieces of organic produce if you wish, but focus on your portion control and nutritional balance, instead of buzzwords.

Fad Diets are Fakes

The Misconception:

You read about it in a celebrity magazine or a coworker says her sister swears by it — a brand-new diet that is going to make the pounds melt away. It sounds simple and practical — you eat only water-based fruits and vegetables or drink an ultra-cleansing lemonade concoction or (even better!) you substitute cookies for two meals a day. This isn't like those other diets! Doctor so-and-so promises you'll drop those troublesome 10 pounds by the end of the week.

The reality is, any diet that makes promises to you using buzzwords like "revolutionary" or "miracle" isn't going to work — or be good for you. Losing weight isn't a quick process, it's a number's game — calories burned versus how many calories ingested.

We all know it takes 3,500 calories burned to lose one pound, thus it's practically impossible to lose 10 pounds in a week. Consider this: Even contestants on the reality weight-loss show *The Biggest Loser*, who are all severely overweight, work out 4 to 6 hours a day, and eat an extremely calorie-restricted diet, scarcely lose 10 pounds a week. So is it logical to think a "miracle" vegetable juice is going to help you do the same?

Also, beware of celebrity-touted diets, which usually lack nutritional considerations and employ extreme calorie restriction. Diets that use the buzzwords "Hollywood" or "celebrity" are always going to be extreme, unhealthy, and more of the impossible get-thin-quick concept. Consider that celebrities are often trying to drop a few pounds for a fashion shoot or to squeeze into a dress at an awards show — but this weight is usually water weight and is gained back immediately after the event. So just because supermodel Heidi Klum says she drank vinegar before each meal to suppress her appetite and lose her baby weight, doesn't mean it makes any sense — or works. And naturally, it isn't a permanent solution.

> Any diet that makes promises to you using buzzwords like "revolutionary" or "miracle" isn't going to work — or be good for you.

The Way to Lose Weight:

Fad diets aren't a lifestyle, they're a quick fix, and even then, many won't give you any results. And the ones that do aren't healthy. It isn't smart or wise to eat nothing but grapefruit or cereal for two meals of the day. You won't be getting the energy and nutrients you need, you'll feel sluggish, and you'll put the weight right back on when you're done with the fad diet.

Don't get trapped on the dieting rollercoaster. You'll be exhausted, discouraged and still not near your target weight. The way to drop unwanted pounds and keep that weight off permanently is to find a diet that works for you on a long-term, day-to-day basis. Whether that means eating 6 small meals a day, limiting your carbohydrates, or shrinking your portion sizes, steer clear of fad diets that employ too-good-to-be-true buzzwords.

When you read health magazines, pay little attention to ads for fad diets or articles on celebrity weight loss and look for the "real reader success stories." These men and women have generally lost weight in a healthy way and have continued to keep it off. These are the diets and workout tips to model yourself after.

Is "Low-Fat" Making You Fat?

The Misconception:

When grocery shopping, you scour the packaging of tasty snacks and foods, such as pretzels, granola bars, yogurt and muffins, for the magical words "low fat" and "fat free." You perk up when a jug of apple juice displays that it is "naturally fat free" and applaud yourself for choosing the "reduced-fat" peanut butter. When you're checking out, you grab a Three Musketeers bar — no need to give up chocolate because this candy bar boasts 45 percent less fat than others. And Ranch dressing can still stay in your diet too, right? Just get the low-fat version. And yet, with a pantry full of these "diet and weight-loss" foods, why aren't you losing weight? Why do you find yourself hungry and frustrated at the end of the day?

Your biggest mistake is in not reading the nutrition labels on these products carefully. If you were to take a closer look, you would see that these low-fat and fat-free items are packed with sugar or high-fructose corn syrup, artificial flavoring or coloring, and chemical preservatives.

Fat-free bakery products are still just desserts in disguise, packed with butter and sugar. Snacks like pretzels and fat-free cookies offer zero nutritional value. They're nothing but empty calories masquerading as "diet-friendly." A reduced-fat candy bar is still a candy bar! A Three Musketeers Bar, even with its airy nougat filling, still contains a diet-denting 260 calories and 40 grams of sugar. And as for reduced-fat peanut butter or salad dressing — check the labels more closely and you'll see these creamy condiments contain more sugar and as many calories as the full-fat versions.

> Here's the real kicker: Dieters actually eat *more* when presented with low-fat products, which have the same or more calories than their full-fat counterparts.

And when you see products like juice boasting that they are "naturally fat free," you should laugh. While fruit doesn't contain fat, most of these drinks contain very small amounts of actual fruit juice and are jam-packed with sugar. Apple juice is notoriously bad: one serving can contain nearly 30 grams of sugar, which is 10 percent of your total daily value of carbohydrates, as well. Again, empty calories in a tiny serving. And buyer beware of juices that brag to have "no sugar added." Generally this means the product had plenty of sugar to begin with, such as cranberry juice blends, another sweet drink that will sabotage your weight-loss efforts.

Glossing over nutrition labels is ignoring the reality of these products, but here's the real kicker: Recent studies have shown that dieters actually eat *more* when presented with low-fat products, which generally have the same or more calories than their full-fat counterparts.

A report called "Can Low Fat Nutrition Labels Lead to Obesity," published in the *Journal of Marketing Research*, offered a dose of reality as to why so many overweight people don't lose a single pound from eating low-fat or fat-free foods. The study found that both normal-weight and overweight participants ate more when presented with a low-fat option of a nutrient-poor and calorie-rich snack food. Additionally, they found that overweight participants were more inclined than normal-weight people to overindulge. Why? The study contends that low-fat food labels increase consumption because they decrease guilt and give the false perception that you can eat more of the item. And it seemed that this was particularly true for overweight subjects.

In a portion of this study, participants were invited to

a university open house and two gallon-size bowls of M&M's were set out, one labeled "New Colors of Regular M&M's" and the other labeled "New 'Low-Fat' M&M's" (although no such low-fat product currently exists). As expected, participants ate more M&M's (28.4 percent more!) when they were labeled as low fat than when they were labeled as regular. Furthermore, overweight participants took 16 percent more M&M's than normal-weight participants. While all participants increased their consumption, overweight subjects ate an average of 90 additional calories more of the candies labeled as "low fat."

The Way to Lose Weight:

Naturally, not all low-fat and fat-free products are bad. Low-fat plain yogurt, for instance, can be a great substitute for high-fat sour cream or mayo in recipes, dips and on baked potatoes. And while not all low-fat cheeses are created equal (some are pretty tasteless), products like Laughing Cow Light Cheese Wedges are healthy and delicious as a spread, dip or melted into a sauce.

When you're opting for the reduced-fat versions of spreads like peanut butter and jelly, look for the brands with less sugar and more natural ingredients. Natural peanut butter has heart-healthy monounsaturated fats and doesn't include the hydrogenated oils, sweeteners and extra salt of other peanut butters. You'll notice the label on natural peanut butter includes only two ingredients: peanuts and salt! Natural peanut butter is a great food for losing weight because it maintains blood-sugar levels and has fiber to keep you feeling full longer. Sugar-free or low-sugar fruit spreads are a great option for when you want something sweet, naturally fat-free and low-calorie. You'll hardly notice the difference in taste between a low-sugar and regular jar of preserves, but you'll be saving 50 calories and 12 grams of sugar per serving!

> If you were to take a closer look, you would see that these low-fat and fat-free items are packed with sugar or high-fructose corn syrup, artificial flavoring or coloring, and chemical preservatives.

If you are able to include snacks in your diet plan, remember that people, especially overweight people, tend to eat more of a low-fat snack than a regular one. This is particularly true if the snack comes in a large bag or container where a serving isn't obvious. Watch out for bags of chips, trail mix, granola or candies that claim to be low-fat, because you're in serious danger of overeating. Instead, manage your calorie and fat intake by choosing snacks like low-fat popcorn or crackers, prepackaged in 100-calorie pouches. You won't be tempted to dive back in for more just because the label reads "low fat."

In the end, low-fat and fat-free claims can be tricky and misleading and studies show they mess with your mind. Don't fall for these buzzwords and assume these products are healthy or will help you lose weight. Losing weight is about reducing your calorie count, eating healthy portions, and stabilizing your blood-sugar levels, none of which can be accomplished with high-sugar items, even if they do have zero grams of fat. The very best way to be sure you're getting the vitamins and nutrients you need without all the fat? Eat fresh, naturally low-fat and fat-free fruits, veggies and whole grains. The fewer ingredients the better and you can't get more natural than chomping on a crisp apple or a handful of sugar snap peas.

Once you start including fresh produce and whole grains in your diet more often, a box of preservative-filled fat-free cookies will look out of place in your cupboards. And as you watch the pounds finally come off, you won't crave the added sugar and empty carbohydrates in the slightest.

"Heart Healthy" Wine, Chocolate and Nuts Require Moderation

The Misconception:

No doubt you've heard that chocolate, wine and nuts can have health benefits, such as preventing heart disease and cancer. You've probably heard the words "flavanols," "antioxidants" and "healthy fats" thrown around. Sounds great, right? You can eat a bag of peanuts at the ballgame, chocolate cake after dinner, and a bottle of wine and improve your health!

Unfortunately, only red wine, some dark chocolate and certain types of nuts have viable benefits, all of which can be met with other, much less caloric foods. Only people who are already healthy and at a stable weight should feel comfortable including wine, chocolate and nuts in their diets.

For people like you who are struggling with weight loss, or health problems like diabetes, it doesn't make sense to add calories and fat to your diet. An antioxidant-rich Dove dark chocolate bar, for instance, contains 190 calories per serving! A 5-ounce glass of red wine has the same amount of antioxidants as dark chocolate; however, each glass also has 120 calories.

In reality, the free radical-fighting antioxidants found in chocolate, cocoa, and red wine are also found naturally in tea, beans and all types of berries, minus the calories and fat.

While studies have shown that people who include nuts in their diets often have lower risk of heart disease, nuts are also very calorie-dense, much of which is from fat. Nuts are only beneficial if they are eaten in careful moderation and do not significantly contribute to your daily calorie count. Unfortunately, because nuts come in large tins and bags, it is just too easy to snack on them by the handful and wreak havoc on your diet.

The Way to Lose Weight:

Like any indulgence — and red wine, chocolate and nuts should be seen as indulgences, not a normal part of your daily diet plan — these foods must be eaten in moderation or they will keep you from losing weight. Buzzwords like "antioxidants" are flying around right now, from the purported benefits of green tea to the Brazilian acai berry.

However, when trying to shed extra pounds, your top considerations should be your intake of calories and fat. Don't fall into the diet trap of thinking, *I can have this chocolate cake — it's good for me.* You're simply cheating yourself out of losing weight.

Dark chocolate can be a fine luxury when eaten in small quantities. Allowing yourself a small indulgence from time to time can keep you on track with your diet because you won't feel deprived. Buy a bar of dark chocolate, but make sure it includes health-benefiting flavanols (many bars are stripped of the flavanols during production, because they give chocolate a bitter taste). Break the bar up into pieces so you get a few bites of chocolate each time, and don't make it a daily habit.

> The free radical-fighting antioxidants found in chocolate, cocoa, and red wine are also found naturally in tea, beans and all types of berries, minus the calories and fat.

As for red wine, men should have no more than 2 alcoholic drinks a day, and one for women, and you should avoid wine and other alcohol if you have diabetes or risk of breast cancer. Know that white wine won't give you the same benefits, because the antioxidant come from the grape skin, which is removed at the start of the process in white wine. And be aware of how drinking affects your eating habits — many people associate wine with food and report that alcohol stimulates their appetite. If a glass of red wine causes you to overeat, the health benefits are clearly negated.

Dark chocolate can be a fine luxury when eaten in small quantities. Allowing yourself a small indulgence can keep you from feeling deprived.

Know that not all nuts are created equal! Good nuts include almonds, walnuts, peanuts and pistachios. Not-so-good nuts, such as macadamias, pecans and Brazil nuts, are high in fat and calories. Because all nuts are calorie-dense, stick to about an ounce of nuts, which equals 160 to 200 calories.

NutHealth.org lists the following as the number of nuts per serving:

- Almonds: 20-24
- Cashews: 16-18

- Macadamias: 10-12
- Brazil nuts: 6-8
- Hazelnuts: 18-20
- Pecans: 18-20 halves
- Pistachios: 45-47
- Pine Nuts: 150-157
- Walnuts: 8-11 halves

Nuts make an easy, crunchy snack, just make sure you always count them out into snack-size baggies. Never try to ration while eating from a jar or bag of nuts — you'll surely overdo it. And be smart: Pass on anything honey-roasted, candied, oil-roasted, or covered in chocolate or yogurt. Raw, unsalted, unroasted nuts are the ones that will make you feel full and satisfied while keeping your calories down. In the right portions, they can be part of a successful weight-loss plan.

Fooling Yourself
by Eating "Fresh"

The Misconception:

Don't believe everything you read: The word "fresh" is just another buzzword used by food manufacturers for emotive appeal — that is, to give you the warm, fuzzy feeling that their product will be good for you.

Every few years, the FDA has come down on different manufacturers who use the word "fresh" in a misleading way. The FDA's standards are based upon what they feel consumers believe the word to mean. Generally speaking, "fresh" indicates juice not from concentrate, products without preservatives, unprocessed fruits and vegetables, and recently baked goods without preservatives.

Why all the debate over the word? The FDA and manufacturers believe that one single word gives those products a decided marketing advantage, proving that people are falling for "fresh" left and right.

Case in point: A West Coast grocery chain that uses

the word "fresh" in their name carries a variety of pre-packaged sandwiches, salads and other meals. While the store markets their meals as artificial color and flavor and trans fat-free, a closer look at the labels reveals that their cranberry and bleu cheese salad has more than 800 calories and their egg salad sandwich contains over 80

> "Fresh" is just another buzzword used by food manufacturers to give you the warm, fuzzy feeling that their product will be good for you.

grams of fat! In fact, you would be hard-pressed to find a pre-made salad or sandwich with less than 600 calories. So while these meals are in fact made "fresh" daily, and "fresh" is right in the store's name, the word itself does not indicate anything is healthy.

Another such example is juice, which often boasts that it is "fresh-squeezed." However, juice, especially apple and grape, are chock full of sugar, natural and added, as well. One 8-ounce glass of juice typically has 150 calories or more.

While "fresh" may indicate a croissant that was baked that morning as opposed to a stale one, the word itself doesn't say anything about a food item's nutritional content or its ability to help you slim down.

The Way to Lose Weight:

Don't be fooled by fresh! Instead of a fat-packed, mayo-heavy tuna salad from your "fresh" neighborhood store, you would be much better served making your own salad from raw ingredients in the produce department and using a light dressing. Fruits and vegetables encompass the true meaning of "fresh."

Whole, raw fruits and vegetables encompass the true meaning of "fresh."

Skip the sugary juice and try calorie-free unsweetened iced tea or water flavored with lemon, orange or cucumber slices. Curious about "no sugar added" juice, such as grape or cherry? All that means is that the fruit contains enough natural sugar that it doesn't need more to sweeten it. It may be "fresh," but it also contains as many calories from sugar as a can of soda.

"Fresh" baked goods are still made with butter, oil and fat. An air-filled puff pastry or sticky bun will sabotage your calorie count for the day right from the start, despite what time of morning it was made. Breeze by the bakery aisle in favor of high-fiber cereal or oatmeal with a side of real fruit.

Above all, stop eating blindly and start reading food labels. "Fresh," like "natural" and "organic," is just a buzzword used by manufacturers hoping to get a leg up on other products. Buzzwords appeal to our culture's desire for a quick fix — don't bother to read the nutritional content, just grab the package that claims to be "fresh." Consumers want the healthy appeal of "fresh," "all-natural" or "green" products, but they often don't want to take the time to think about what's really in what they're eating. Don't be fooled by marketing. By taking a few minutes to look over the labels on the foods you buy, you can make informed decisions about what you're putting into your body.

And remember, the fewer ingredients in something, the more fresh it really is, so stick to a whole banana (ingredients: one) instead of a banana smoothie or banana muffin.

Meal Replacement Bars and Drinks Aren't the Answer

The Misconception:

The words "meal replacement" conjure up images of quick and simple weight loss, without cooking a meal or making any tough food decisions. You don't even have to chew! Meal replacement shakes and bars helped you slim down quickly before a beach vacation, so you turn to them in place of one or two meals a day when you need to drop a few pounds fast. You're just not sure why they don't help you keep the weight off permanently, which is your ultimate goal.

The other puzzling thing is why some meal replacement drinks, shakes and bars taste so much better than others! With the vast different in taste and texture, you aren't sure which to choose.

Well, the truth is, meal replacements just aren't going to be a permanent solution for the majority of people. You might drop 5 pounds for your vacation — enough to feel confident in your swimsuit — but the second you abandon the drinks, the weight comes right back in a hurry. Most people want taste and variety from their food; thus, it isn't realistic to eat Special K cereal or drink Slim Fast smoothies twice a day for much longer than a week or two. Not to mention the cost! At $15 or more a week, these items can get expensive.

Another reason meal replacement drinks, shakes and smoothies don't work? They don't fulfill many dieters. Much of eating is mental, and research has shown that people need to chew in order to feel full and satisfied. Liquid meals don't provide that opportunity, so dieters are left wanting to eat again, despite the fact that they have ingested over 200 calories.

As for meal replacement bars, many are just glorified candy bars. The general rule of thumb for these bars is, the better it tastes, the worse it is for you. The bars that taste best generally contain cheap simple sugars, such as fructose and dextrose, which give a burst of energy

> The meal replacement bars that taste best generally contain cheap simple sugars, such as fructose and dextrose, which give a burst of energy followed by a crash.

Stick to drinks and bars that provide a balanced 40/30/30 or 40/40/20 ratio of carbohydrates, fats, and proteins.

followed by a crash. Other bars are made with sugar alcohols, like glycerine, which give many people an upset stomach, cramps and diarrhea.

Also be wary of bars with heavy carb and calorie counts. A 350-calorie bar with 60 grams of carbs might be appropriate for someone on an intense exercise plan, but not for you, trying to lose weight. There's a reason many of these bars were designed for long-distance cyclists or mountain climbers. You're not peaking Mount Rainier? Then skip a calorie-heavy bar.

The Way to Lose Weight:

While meal replacement bars and drinks are never ideal, they are certainly the better choice when you need nutrition in a hurry and your other option is the drive-thru. Stick to drinks and bars that provide a balanced 40/30/30 or 40/40/20 ratio of carbohydrates, fats, and proteins.

Steer clear of bars with too many simple sugars, which add

empty carbs and don't satiate you over an extended time period. Instead, look for a bar with more fiber, which will make you feel full longer. And stay away from anything that contains partially hydrogenated oils, which are a source of heart-clogging trans fats.

Know that meal replacements are just another diet trend, another quick fix. Don't pretend you can replace two or more meals a day with a bar or drink for the rest of your life. If you want to incorporate meal replacements into your diet plan, stick to only one a day for maintenance once you reach a weight you're comfortable with.

Instead of a bar, shake or drink, try putting together snack-size baggies of healthy, crisp foods like apple slices, celery, snap peas, carrots and bell peppers, which give you a satisfying crunch and remind your body that you're eating *real* food.

Lose V
Get a

eight, Clue!

Chapter 5

Lose Weight, Get a Clue!

Listen up: This is the chapter where we confront all the ridiculous bad habits that make dieters smack their foreheads and say, "Doh!" You may not even be aware that you exhibit some of these behaviors. Others may sound obvious, such as not skipping breakfast or drinking your calories, but you'll see that food culture in the United States is such that you may be totally unaware of your mistakes and misconceptions. For instance, did you know that studies have proven that our perceptions of serving size are highly ineffective and that most people will underestimate the caloric value of a dish by nearly half? Studies have also shown that cooks and restaurants have very little concern for the healthiness of their food and care much more about price point and perceived value (size) of their products. This leaves the responsibility solely to you — to be informed and accountable for your eating choices.

In this chapter you'll get invaluable tools for losing real weight and losing it quickly, including the trick every thin and fit person knows — keeping a food diary. You're not sure if you want to take the time to write down every single thing you eat and drink every day? The proven weight-loss stats should change your mind.

You'll also learn to fix the top mistakes clueless dieters make again and again — the ones that keep nutritionists and diet coaches in business. Skipping meals in hopes of cutting calories or relying on eating huge portions are classic blunders, but do you realize just how much they're contributing to your weight problem? You'll be shocked. Luckily, everything you need to know to make a lifestyle adjustment and stop these bad behaviors is right here in these pages.

This chapter is all about getting clued in to the crazy diet mistakes we make without even realizing it, as well as the boldface lies we tell ourselves that tack on calories, fat, sodium and extra pounds. As long ago as 500 BC, Chinese philosopher Confucius said, "When it is obvious that the goals cannot be reached, don't adjust the goals, adjust the action steps." What you've *been* doing isn't working, so it's time to create a new game plan for slimming down. Being clueless is no longer an excuse for being overweight and obese — now that you have the tools, secrets and knowledge to lose weight, the only thing left to do is put it all into action.

Instant Diet Makeover Tips:

▸ Drink plenty of water each day. Often we think we are hungry when our body is sending us signals that we are actually thirsty or dehydrated. Water also enables your body to work effectively at burning stored fat.

▸ Get lots of sleep. Lack of sleep can lead to an increase in appetite, especially cravings for fatty and sugary foods.

▸ Choose carbs wisely. Eat a 100-calorie apple versus eating a 100-calorie serving of chips.

▸ Heat up your food. Foods served hot can be more satiating, so you are likely to eat less.

▸ Keep healthy snacks in your kitchen. That way, when you have the urge to munch on something, you will have better choices on hand.

▸ Look for local or online weight-loss support communities where you can share your story, get tips, and ask for support from other dieters.

▸ Celebrate your success every day. Be proud of what you have accomplished and continue to envision the future you.

All Calories Count,
So Start Keeping Track

The Misconception:

You don't need to keep a food diary, because you have an honest, accurate sense of what you eat each day. The occasional burger or snack can't really make *that* big of a difference in your waistline. Well then, why aren't you losing weight?

The reality is, eating half a bag of chips or hitting up the drive thru, even occasionally, is a big deal and is preventing you from dropping unwanted pounds. Losing weight is a simple equation — burn more calories than you ingest — and how do you expect to do that without writing down everything you eat?

For one, dieters often have absolutely no idea how many calories or grams of fat are in what they eat if the item doesn't have a food label. Think about it: Can you accurately guess how many calories are in your favorite turkey sandwich from the deli? You might estimate 400 or 500 calories. Actually, if it's served on cheesy or oily bread, like focaccia, or is dressed up with mayo or several slices of cheese, you could be looking at 800 calories or more! That is half of some people's caloric intake for the entire day!

> Keeping a daily food diary will not only keep you accountable for what you eat, it will reveal correlations between food and your mood and energy levels.

Additionally, people tend to have generous and selective memories when it comes to what they have eaten. How many times have you "forgotten" about a half of a muffin, a handful of crackers, or finishing your child's cookie? Studies have shown again and again that dieters must record everything they eat in order to hold themselves accountable.

In fact, in 2008 the *American Journal of Preventive Medicine* followed 1,700 overweight or obese men and women (the average weight was 212 pounds) who were following an exercise and diet plan. The subjects who did not record what they ate lost 9 pounds. However, those who did keep a food journal lost twice as much weight or an average of 18 pounds.

The Way to Lose Weight:

Start keeping a food diary and record every meal, snack and drink you have each day. Your diary should also include space to record your mood and energy levels, as well as any exercise you do. Try *The Ultimate Pocket Diet Journal*, one of the best-selling diet journals on the market, or simply get a blank notebook.

Also, you need to keep a calorie-counting tool handy for when you dine out and items don't offer nutritional information. A great book is the portable, pocket-size *Complete Calorie, Fat & Carb Counter*, which provides calories, fat, carbs, fiber and protein for menu items from more than 500 fast-food chains, restaurants, and popular food brands.

Keeping a daily food diary will not only keep you accountable for what you eat and drink, it will reveal correlations between the food you eat and your mood and energy levels. While it's intuitive that eating a huge lunch makes you sluggish in the afternoon, it has a greater impact when you see it on paper. And when you realize, *Gosh, I ate 900 calories today at lunch*, you'll think twice about getting that fully loaded burrito the next time. Participants in the *American Journal of Preventive Medicine* study reported that they found keeping a food diary to be "enlightening."

You will also find less urge to binge or eat sugary foods because you will be answering to your food diary later, and you won't be able to pretend you didn't eat those three mini Snickers bars. Day by day, your food diary will help you cut calories until you start losing weight steadily. You will see how eliminating just a few hundreds calories — one less soda here, one less dessert there — will jumpstart your weight loss.

A food diary will also help you gauge your progress as you work toward a diet plan you can live with. It will be very encouraging to look back over the weeks and months and see how your portion control and food choices have been improving and how you are finally losing weight.

There is no reason to give up your food diary once healthier eating becomes your lifestyle. Many people who stop keeping track of what they eat find they start cheating on their diets again right away. Writing down what you eat and drink means you are in control of your weight and have the power to adjust your diet as needed.

Bad Portion Control is Out of Control

The Misconception:

Do you know what a single serving is for your favorite foods, such as pasta, chicken, rice, oatmeal, yogurt and more? No need for annoying measuring cups or a food scale, if the packaging says that ½ cup or 6 ounces is a serving you can just eyeball the correct amount. A handful here and a scoop there ... that looked like a tablespoon, right? Wrong. Studies have proven that people are terribly inaccurate when it comes to eyeballing portions.

A study referenced in the *Journal of Marketing Research* showed that consumers' perceptions of serving size are highly unreliable and can unknowingly vary as much as 20 percent. Another study showed that consumers vastly underestimate the caloric content of the foods they eat. In a 2006 study, researchers asked consumers to estimate the number of calories in different fast food meals. Most participants estimated 700 to 800 calories for these meals — about half of the actual amount.

Another study of the factors that lead to over-consumption, published in the *Journal of Consumer Research* in 2008, found that a concept called "extremeness aversion" also contributes to bad portion control, overeating and obesity. Extremeness aversion is the tendency for individuals to avoid the smallest and largest sizes and order the middle size — no matter how large. According to Kathryn M. Sharpe, Richard Staelin and Joel Huber, authors of the study, this concept has gradually led retailers to offer larger and larger portions and consumers to choose larger and larger portions. You may have noticed that businesses like movie theaters and fast food restaurants have begun to inflate the sizes of highly caloric items like popcorn, fries and soft drinks. The 2008 study showed that if a fast food restaurant originally offered 21-ounce, 16-ounce and 12-ounce options for soft drinks, most consumers would rule out the large and small sizes and choose the middle size, 16 ounces. However, when the restaurant eliminated the 12-ounce drink, consumers would choose the 21-ounce drink, because the 16-ounce drink they preferred earlier was now the smallest size, or the extreme, making it less desirable. The study of extremeness aversion contended that consumers still want the 16-ounce drink, and businesses could help Americans trim their waistlines by eliminating the largest sizes and bringing back the smaller sizes.

So, not only are consumers' perceptions of correct serving

size highly inaccurate, but businesses are constantly increasing their portion sizes to reflect the concept of "extremeness aversion," in which consumers tend to choose the middle portion size, no matter how unnecessarily large. Worse still, studies demonstrate that people grossly underestimate the number of calories in food! Bottom line: You're eating bad food and way too much of it and not even realizing it. Time to wise up.

The Way to Lose Weight:

Most diet experts agree you can eat most of the foods you love if you exercise portion control. First, that means educating yourself about what one serving of your favorite foods really is!

According to the USDA, one serving equals*:

- 1 slice of whole grain bread
- 1/2 cup of cooked rice or pasta
- 1/2 cup of mashed potatoes
- 3-4 small crackers
- 1 small pancake or waffle
- 2 medium-sized cookies
- 1/2 cup cooked vegetables
- 1/2 cup tomato sauce
- 1 cup lettuce

- 1 small baked potato
- 1 medium apple
- 1/2 grapefruit or mango
- 1/2 cup berries
- 1/3 cup dried fruit or nuts
- 2 tbsp peanut butter
- 1 cup yogurt or milk
- 1 1/2 ounces of cheese
- 1/2 cup dry beans
- 1/2 cup tofu
- 1 chicken breast
- 1 medium pork chop
- 1/4 pound hamburger patty
- 1 tsp butter or margarine

* Keep in mind that certain factors affect food portions, such as the individual's age, gender and activity level.

Now, we've discussed how most people can't eyeball portions without some practice. You won't always have a measuring cup on-hand, and who knows what an ounce of something looks like? Create a system in which you associate the size of a familiar object, like a golf ball or your fist, to serving sizes of your favorite foods.

Here is a list to help you get started, or come up with your own serving-size associations if you like:

- Vegetables or fruit: the size of your fist or a baseball

- Pasta: one handful
- Meat, fish, or poultry: a deck of cards or the size of your palm
- Snacks (chips, pretzels, etc): a cupped handful
- Apple: a baseball
- Potato: a computer mouse
- Bagel: a hockey puck
- Pancake: a CD
- Ice cream: a tennis ball
- Steamed rice: a cupcake wrapper
- Cheese: size of your whole thumb
- Dried fruit or nuts: a golf ball or an egg
- Cereal: a fist
- Dinner roll: a bar of soap
- Peanut butter: a ping pong ball
- Butter or margarine: a postage stamp
- Salad dressing: a ping pong ball

After some time, you will be able to recognize correct portions just by how they fill up a plate, bowl or pan. You'll also learn that the brain — and stomach! — can be tricked into thinking you've eaten more than you have, allowing you to enjoy smaller portions. One trick that can help when you're eating at home is using smaller plates, bowls, glasses and spoons. Think about it: If you're using a large dinner plate, you're more inclined to fill it completely with spaghetti and meatballs — and eat the whole plate of food. But if you fill smaller dishware and silverware, it gives the impression that there is more food or drink, so your brain will report that you're full and satisfied from a smaller portion.

Also, your sense of satiation is very visual. If you set baskets or pans food out on the table, you are simply encouraging yourself to take seconds. Serve yourself a reasonable portion size while you're in the kitchen, then put the rest of the food away for leftovers. This way you won't be tempted to take more of anything. Savor and appreciate each bite of food. Busy yourself with dishes and cleaning up your cooking space — this gives your brain a chance to register that your body is full, and you won't feel the need to grab another dinner roll or helping of potatoes.

When you're eating out of a container, there is also a tendency to feel like you haven't eaten enough to satisfy you. If you take the food out of the packaging your brain will register just how much you're really eating. A yogurt may not look like much in its packaging, but you'll discover its contents actually fill a bowl. And how many times have you gotten to the bottom of a 100-calorie snack pack and commented, "There were only four cookies in there!" If you pour them out ahead of time, your brain has a chance to register that you are, in fact, eating a full handful of small cookies, which is a healthy portion.

We all know that portion control is much easier when we're eating at home. At home we can regulate how much we put on a plate, whereas at a restaurant, portions are often two and even three times the size of what we'd serve ourselves. A huge part of losing weight and keeping it off is learning to identify a healthy portion when dining out. Start by always opting for the smallest portion size available. Many restaurants offer a "bistro size" or "lunch portion" of their salads and entrées. This portion size will leave you happy and full at 99 percent of restaurants. Or, order an appetizer version of a full entrée, such a veggie quesadilla or steamed mussels. When you find yourself wondering, "Will the half salad be enough?" remember that restaurants very often inflate portion sizes in order to charge more. Cut calories and save money by opting for the smaller portion.

Another smart dieters' trick is to ask for a doggie bag or to-go container as soon as your entrée touches down on the table. Determine an appropriate portion and set aside the rest for leftovers. When the entire meal stays on your plate, you are constantly tempted to keep eating and eating until your plate is bare. Think about how many times you've thought, *Well, I've eaten two-thirds of this meal already, so I may as well finish the rest.* Store half your meal out of sight and feel content when the plate is empty.

Skipping Meals Isn't Helping You Slim Down

The Misconception:

Since losing weight is a simple mathematical calculation of ingesting fewer calories than you burn, you figure skipping a meal or two should help you get thin. Perhaps your mindset is that if you stay busy at work or with your family you won't feel the need to eat and you can save hundreds of calories.

Plus, cutting calories by skipping meals seems much easier than eliminating the foods you love, like burgers and fries. You think, *I skipped lunch so I can have a second helping of macaroni and cheese with dinner.*

Your delusion is two-fold. First, cutting calories here by skipping lunch, only to spend them there with a cheesy side dish isn't really cutting back on anything, now is it.

Second, and much more important, skipping meals is never the way to cut calories or lose weight. In fact, quite the opposite is true and you may actually gain weight. Food is fuel for your body and when you skip a meal your system goes into starvation mode. Your metabolism slows down to conserve energy and your body prepares to store fat during your next meal.

Worse still, most people end up bingeing the next time they do eat, overcompensating for the skipped meal. When you skip a

> Try having three small meals and two or three healthy snacks to keep your metabolism working continuously and avoid blood sugar surges and crashes.

meal, your blood sugar drops steadily, leading to dizziness and hunger pangs, causing you to overeat. Many dieters will skip meals all day, eating only a small piece of fruit or a light snack, only to find they are ravenous by bedtime, the worst time of the day to eat.

The Way to Lose Weight:

Don't confuse your body by skipping meals; instead, eat small portions throughout the day. Try having three small meals and two or three healthy snacks throughout your day. This keeps your metabolism revved and working

Skipping meals is never the way to cut calories or lose weight. In fact, quite the opposite is true and you may actually gain weight.

continuously and avoids blood sugar surges and crashes.

It is especially important to eat breakfast — and no, a cup of coffee isn't breakfast. Whole grains, oats, peanut butter, fruit, low-fat yogurt, and eggs are all good ways to start your day. They get your metabolism kicking and provide a boost of energy that should last a few hours.

Try to eat every three or four hours and choose nutritious foods — light cheese and whole grain crackers, salads, hummus and vegetables, peanut butter on whole wheat toast, baked fish and chicken — and you won't overindulge at any one meal.

Beware of Drive-By Snacking

The Misconception:

Food is often presented in a way that makes it seem casual, easy and friendly — a bowl of M&M's on the secretary's desk at work, kiosks of samples at Costco, attractive hors d'oeuvres at a party, or a tray of bite-size tasters at the coffee shop. Without thinking, you grab a handful of candy each time you walk to your desk. At a party, you take something off every tray of hors d'oeuvres that comes around. As you chat with friends, "Ooh, I'll try that," becomes, "Sure, I'll have another." Soon you have a pile of cocktail napkins and crumbs in your hand. And by the time you leave the club store, you've eaten enough sample-size snacks to constitute an entire meal. (Isn't that half the fun of going to Costco anyway?) However, when it comes time to tally your calories for the day, these drive-by snacking incidents are mysteriously forgotten, leaving you to wonder why the weight isn't coming off.

You have fooled yourself into believing that drive-by snacking — a few bites here, a few bites there — doesn't constitute a full snack or meal. But consider this: Would you eat a jumbo-size bag of M&M's in one sitting? No? Unfortunately, grabbing handfuls of M&M's throughout your workday equates to the same thing.

And think of it this way: At a party, if the hors d'oeuvres weren't being brought around by servers but were set out on a table, would you pile your plate high or would you know to take only two or three small samples?

When it comes time to tally your calories for the day, these drive-by snacking incidents are mysteriously forgotten.

Unfortunately, our brains often trick us into thinking that eating something bite-size means it's better for us than eating the same food in its full size. But this is only true if you eat just a few bite-size pieces! And studies have shown that small treats, such as mini-cookies, actually lead people to eat more than they would if the cookies were full-size. If you wouldn't eat a whole cheese Danish, why eat four samples at the coffee shop? You're not doing your waistline any favors, and you're actually doing yourself a double disservice by pretending those calories don't count.

The Way to Lose Weight:

By nature, drive-by snacking is mindless, which is why we let those calories slide when we take a mental tally of what we ate that day. Always eat consciously. At a party, be wary of the hand-to-mouth motion while you're chatting with friends. And for heaven's sake — you don't need to accept every time a waiter comes by offering hors d'oeuvres.

Hors d'oeuvres are always rich and fatty in order to pack lots of flavor in a small bite. Items like filled puff pastries, crab cakes, deviled eggs, bacon-wrapped shrimp, and creamy dips are popular and each has a ton of calories. You could be consuming 100 calories or more per bite! Instead, fill up on crunchy crudités (raw veggies), shrimp cocktail, or smoked salmon. And never, ever feel bad about saying "No thank you" more than half the time the server comes by. The hors d'oeuvres at the party *will* get eaten — just not by you.

> Losing weight comes from holding yourself accountable — including your guilty pleasures, little indulgences and bad habits.

Stopping drive-by snacking also means making smart tradeoffs — again, being conscious that these calories do count. For instance, if you like the samples at the store, be picky about the ones you try, and don't just grab every single one. And if you have five samples, leave one thing off your dinner plate to compensate. If you try a few samples of the new pastries at Starbucks, tell yourself that is your dessert quota for the day.

Finally, take away the opportunity for temptation by avoiding situations where calorie-packed treats are easy to grab. Don't post up by the hors d'oeuvres table at a party. Stand away from the entrance to the kitchen so you're not the first guest servers with fresh trays of snacks see. Never have bowls of candy, snack mix or chocolate on your desk or around your home. If your officemate always puts out Hershey's Kisses, avoid her desk! If you do have to linger in her area, be actively aware of the treats. It's the unconscious hand-to-mouth nature of drive-by snacking that tacks on hundreds of unwanted calories.

And be sure to include all your drive-by snacking in your food diary. Losing weight comes from holding yourself accountable — and that includes your guilty pleasures, little indulgences and bad habits. Not even a bite of a cookie should slip by!

Get Smart About Frozen Diet Meals

The Misconception:

In an attempt to resist the lure of the drive-thru or the lunchtime buffet line, many dieters turn to lunches and dinners from the freezer section as a means to lose weight. They hope to benefit from a low-calorie meal in a portion-controlled package.

Unfortunately, the upside of frozen diet meals, which is that they are low in calories, is also one of their main drawbacks. The majority of diet meals contain between 200 and 350 calories. For most people, this isn't enough to leave them satisfied. These meals usually contain little fiber to help fill you up, and so after eating you may feel hungry again right away.

Additionally, frozen meals are packed with preservatives and sodium — up to 1,800 milligrams of sodium, in fact. For most people, this is practically their entire sodium intake for the day, and for people with high blood pressure, who should stick to less than 1500 milligrams, it's more than a day's worth. Unfortunately, it's the sodium content that keeps the sauces and vegetables in frozen meals tasting good.

> Since satiation can be very visual, take the meal out of the package and eat it from a plate.

When it comes to vegetables in frozen diet meals, many are lacking. Some options, such as macaroni and cheese, don't pretend to offer any servings of vegetables at all. And the products that do state how many servings of vegetables they contain aren't always accurate.

One article, published in the *Nutrition Action Healthletter*, found that many of the frozen meals they tested contained half or even a third of the "full cup of vegetables" they claimed to include. Thus, don't pretend that you're loading up on healthy veggies by eating one Lean Cuisine.

The Way to Lose Weight:

One nice thing about frozen diet meals is they take the guesswork out of portion control. Studies have proven again and again that Americans are terrible at estimating a correct portion size, so having a prepackaged dinner can keep you from overdoing it. However, the small size can also be what keeps you from feeling satisfied after eating a frozen diet meal. One look at that tiny box and you start wondering what else there is to eat.

Since satiation can be very visual, one trick is to take the meal out of the package and put it on a plate after you've heated it up. For one, it looks like more food when it's out of the box, and when you eat on a real plate with real utensils you feel more like you've gotten a complete meal. You won't be tempted to have a snack in 30 minutes.

If you like the convenience of frozen diet meals, try making a large batch of fresh food that can be divided into servings, frozen and reheated later.

One nice thing about these meals is that you will get used to seeing what a low-calorie portion size actually looks like, both in the package and on a plate. Learning to eyeball proper portions is a huge step toward eating the right amounts to lose weight.

As mentioned earlier, the portions of vegetables in frozen diet meals can be rather meager. Ideally, you should be getting between 5 and 11 half-cup servings of vegetables and fruits a day. Try meeting this quota by supplementing a low-calorie frozen meal with an extra ½-cup serving of fresh veggies, such as steamed broccoli.

One nice thing about frozen meals is that you will get used to seeing what a low-calorie portion size actually looks like, both in the package and on a plate.

Adding your own fresh extras to these meals is the best way to make them taste great while still being healthy. Eat a whole wheat roll or a small salad on the side. Or, add a spoonful of salsa or hot sauce, which are very flavorful while being low-calorie and fat-free.

When choosing frozen diet meals, look for ones with low saturated fat and a balance of veggies and lean protein. Toss in a low-calorie vegetable-topped pizza or panini as a treat. And always choose the meals that are low in sodium, about 500 milligrams or less. Low-sodium options will prevent you from feeling bloated and gaining water weight and help keep your blood pressure stable.

And you don't have to sacrifice taste for health. Amy's vegetarian, organic products are favorites of many frozen meal-lovers and offer an extensive low-sodium line. Most meals made by Organic Bistro contain more than 30 grams of protein, plus unprocessed organic ingredients mean they're packed with taste without added salt and artificial flavorings. Kashi and Lean Cuisine's Spa Cuisine line both include lots of filling fiber into their tasty, healthy dinners using ingredients like whole wheat noodles.

While fresh is always better than frozen, many busy people enjoy the fact that frozen meals save them time. They don't have to plan a menu, do extensive grocery shopping, cook, or even leave their desks for lunch. If you like the efficiency and convenience of frozen diet meals, try taking one evening or weekend afternoon to make a large batch of fresh food that can be divided into servings, frozen and reheated later. Soup, chili, and vegetarian lasagna are just a few great options that can be made in healthy ways. Store each portion in an airtight container, freeze and enjoy for up to three months.

Don't Miss (or Mess Up) the Most Important Meal of the Day

The Misconception:

Even though you probably just wanted to sleep in for a few more minutes, your mom always woke you up for a bowl of oatmeal or eggs and toast before school, because "breakfast is the most important meal of the day." But now that you're a busy adult, there's no time for a leisurely, balanced breakfast on the weekdays and many weekends. Breakfast often falls by the wayside or consists of a cup of coffee. Like many people, you may claim you just aren't hungry in the mornings. Skipping breakfast is extremely common.

Or, you may be a breakfast lover (Americans, especially, are known for our big breakfasts; think, Denny's Grand Slam). On workdays you generally don't have time to cook a full breakfast, so you pick up a breakfast sandwich or breakfast burrito at a fast-food restaurant or when you stop to get your morning coffee. These types of meals are quick and simple to eat while you're in your car and on the go.

However, skipping breakfast, or eating the wrong things, sets you up for an entire day of bad eating and feeling sluggish and slow.

If you're skipping breakfast you're really missing out on all the benefits to your health, weight and even productivity the first meal of the day can have. The term "breakfast" literally means a "break" from a "fast." Think about it: You probably eat your last meal of the day between 6 and 8 p.m., then go to sleep and don't have an opportunity to eat again for about 12 hours. Your body has been fasting — your metabolism has slowed and your system is storing fat and energy, preparing for the next day. If you skip breakfast and go all the way until noon without eating, you are depriving your body of nutrients and the fuel it needs to produce energy for about 18 hours! Without breakfast, you will have less focus, less oomph and will be less productive. And, have you noticed how when you skip breakfast you find yourself starving by lunchtime, where you overcompensate with a huge meal? Now you know why you spend all afternoon feeling sleepy and lethargic — and why breakfast is so important.

More Americans are eating breakfast than ever before, partly because the benefits have been highly publicized over the years, but also because quick and convenient breakfast options are popping up in new, even unexpected places all the time. From Subway restaurants offering breakfast sandwiches to nearly every fast-food chain incorporating breakfast burritos, bowls and wraps in their menus, retailers are recognizing that breakfast food is a huge money-maker and are seeking to offer it throughout the day. Breakfast is truly the fastest-growing meal of the day; unfortunately, the portion sizes and calorie counts are expanding, as well.

Ever notice how your morning bagel actually makes you feel *hungrier* after you eat it?

Parade Magazine's annual report, "What America Really Eats," found that breakfast is actually becoming the highest-calorie meal of the day for many consumers. That's because breakfast sandwiches and burritos — generally made with bacon, ham, cheese, fried potatoes and eggs — made the top 10 on both men and women's lists of most-ordered menu items last year. In 2007, 20 percent of consumers reported eating breakfast on the go at least three times a week — and unfortunately, a typical drive-thru breakfast sandwich or burrito boasts between 500 and 800 calories. And that's not including the foamy latte or glass of juice you are also probably having. Thus, that meal you're quickly eating while driving to work can bring your daily total to nearly 1,000 calories — and all by 8 a.m.

The Way to Lose Weight:

First, eat breakfast. Duh. It is the most important meal of the day — your mother was right. That's because a balanced breakfast normalizes your body after many hours of rest. Eating breakfast revs your metabolism and gets your body burning calories right away. Without this jumpstart, your body goes into starvation mode and prepares to store fat during your next meal.

Breakfast also stabilizes your blood-sugar levels so you're not starving and woozy by 11 a.m. When you have low blood sugar, you're more inclined to eat a huge lunch, and a fat-filled one at that. In 2009, researchers from the Imperial College of London found that the reward centers of the brain responded greatly to high-calorie, fatty foods at lunchtime in participants who skipped breakfast. On the contrary, the subjects who ate breakfast were far less likely to be enticed by fatty foods.

> Breakfast is becoming the highest-calorie meal of the day for many consumers — breakfast sandwiches and burritos made the top 10 most-ordered menu items last year.

Not to mention how crappy you feel after eating too much at lunch. When you skip a meal in the morning only to overeat in the middle of the day, your body slips into a "food coma" and your afternoon productivity goes to zero.

Not only does breakfast kick-start your metabolism and help you eat a normal portion at lunch, it gives you blood-sugar stability that means more energy and focus for your work. However, not all breakfasts are balanced and healthy, as the 800-calorie breakfast sandwich proves. Too many people start their days with refined carbs. Simply put, refined carbs are items made with sugars and white flour, such as bagels, donuts and muffins. Ever notice how your morning bagel actually makes you feel *hungrier* after you eat it? That's because the body processes refined carbs so quickly that your blood sugar surges. So, you've not only eaten a 450-calorie bagel with cream cheese, you're ready to eat again mid-morning.

A better choice for weight loss? Protein-packed eggs. Case in point: A study from the Pennington Biomedical Research Center showed that participants who ate two eggs for breakfast lost 65 percent more weight than participants who ate a bagel, even though the bagel and the eggs contained an equal number of calories. The egg-eaters also reported feeling more energetic than the participants who ate bagels.

Now, you do need some carbs, but make sure they're complex carbs, such a whole wheat English muffin or oatmeal (without all the sugary toppings). Complex carbs make you feel full and burn directly into energy.

Cereal is also a morning favorite; the *Parade Magazine* study reported that 67 percent of respondents eat cereal for breakfast. Just stay away from cereals marketed to children — the boxes with the cartoon characters and free toys. According to a study from Yale University's Rudd Center for Food Policy and Obesity, breakfast cereals marketed to children contain 85 percent more sugar, 65 percent less fiber, and 60 percent more sodium than those targeted at adults.

A breakfast that balances complex carbs with protein, fiber-filled veggies in an omelet, a piece of fruit, or low-fat dairy is a fantastic way to lose weight and eat with stability from sun-up to sundown. Just be smart and don't pretend that "the most important meal of the day" is a McDonald's Deluxe Breakfast (scrambled eggs, biscuit, sausage patty, hotcakes, hash browns, margarine and syrup that add up to 1,220 calories and 61 grams of fat). That's more like breakfast for your entire carpool!

Look Out for Liquid Calories

The Misconception:

You watch what you eat and you know better than to drink soda (evil!), which is full of sugar and calories. Instead, you like real fruit juice or a smoothie in the mornings, iced tea at lunch, a sports drink during your workout, and a glass or two of wine or beer with dinner. Or, maybe you eat healthy all week so that you can enjoy cocktails and dinner with friends on the weekends. Watching sports usually means beers with the guys on Saturdays or Sundays. But regular soda? Never. So why do you feel like the scale is stuck?

The phrase "drinking your calories" doesn't just refer to drinking soda, but too many dieters believe that switching from Sprite to Sprite Zero means they've done enough to fix their bad habits. Hate to break it to you but fruit juice and smoothies, sweetened tea, sports drinks, energy drinks, protein shakes, and alcohol are all *packed* with calories, sugar and carbs, just like soda, and sometimes more so.

Plus, have you ever looked closely at the labels of your Gatorade, Naked Juice, Arizona Iced Tea or Monster? Most bottled drinks contain more than 1 serving — 2.5 servings per bottle is typical. If you drink the whole bottle, which most people do, you're drinking 200 to 400 calories in just a few gulps.

This misconception is not entirely your fault. Media and advertising have long positioned juice, smoothies and fruit drinks as "healthy." Slews of TV commercials featuring famous pro athletes lead you to believe that sports drinks like Gatorade and Vitamin Water help you stay fit and healthy. The reality is, fruit drinks are often made with very little real fruit and contain lots of added sugar. Soft-serve yogurt, ice cream, sherbet and other dairy products give smoothies their smooth texture while adding sugar, calories and carbs. And unless you actually *are* a pro athlete, or working out as hard as one, you don't need all those empty calories and carbs for energy.

> It's easy to forget about 250 calories when they're in liquid form, but cutting those calories can make a big difference in the amount of weight you lose.

Alcohol is one of those things that can creep up on you and

really sabotage your weight-loss progress. For one, it's easy to say, "I'll just have one drink" and then let one round turn into two or three or more. And many people find themselves unwinding with a cocktail of some sort every night. Many drinkers (typically women) make the mistake of thinking they can build the calories from alcohol into their daily totals, causing them to skip nutritious food in favor of alcohol. Others (typically men) simply drink more when their inhibitions are lowered by alcohol, leading to weight gain.

Consider the approximate calorie counts for these alcoholic drinks:

- Light beer: 100 calories
- Glass of wine: 120 calories
- Regular beer: 150 calories
- Shot: 70 to 100 calories
- Mixed drink: 200 calories
- Blended drink (margarita or piña colada): 400 calories

Now, consider how many hundreds of extra calories you're adding to your daily intake by throwing back a few cocktails.

The real problem with getting so many calories and carbs from liquids is that they don't fill you up, so you wind up eating on top of what you're drinking. Satiation comes from chewing, thus many times a liquid will be ingested unconsciously in just a few gulps, without helping you to feel full and without any thought for the calories you just consumed. It's easy to forget about 250 calories when they're in liquid form, but cutting out 250 calories can make a big difference in the amount of weight you lose.

The Way to Lose Weight:

The good news is drinks are a quick and easy place to cut extra calories to lose more weight. Regular sodas are out — you're on the right track there. But that's not enough to lose weight and keep it off permanently. You need to be acutely aware of everything you're drinking so you're not adding hundreds of empty calories and carbs to your daily intake. Again (scream it from the rooftops!), you need to be keeping a food diary and you need to be recording everything you drink, as well as eat.

Let's start with breakfast: Skip the smoothie unless it's real fruit blended with ice or a small amount of OJ or nonfat plain yogurt for thickness. Smoothies only make a smart breakfast if they keep you full until it's time for your small mid-morning snack. For many people, an all-fruit smoothie just isn't enough to hold them over — and therein lies the problem. You can also add oatmeal, peanut butter or almond butter to smoothies to make them thicker and more filling. Or consider a protein-boost, such as whey powder. In the end, a smoothie is a quick fix when you're in a hurry but not a practical daily breakfast for weight loss. Instead of a smoothie, have real fruit on the side of some whole grains.

If you love fruit juice with breakfast, make sure you're checking the calories and sugar on these beverages. Look for low-calorie or low-sugar versions of your favorite juices. Pour yourself a small glass, which will provide just enough flavor and sweetness to satisfy you, without adding lots of extra calories. And, of course, look for products that are real juice. Avoid anything labeled with the words "drink," "beverage" or "cooler." Fake-juice products, such as the childhood favorite Sunny Delight, list high fructose corn syrup as their top ingredient after water and contain only a tiny amount of real fruit juice.

For lunch, opt for water with lemon or low-calorie iced tea. Just remember to order unsweetened iced tea. Add a squeeze of lemon or orange if need be.

In the evenings and on weekends, the temptation to relax with an alcoholic drink (or several drinks) is high for many people. But there is not much room for alcohol when you're trying to lose weight. And, for people wanting to keep the weight off for a lifetime, you're going to have to seriously limit the amount of booze you drink permanently.

First and foremost, when you drink alcohol, that is what your body processes first, before fat, protein or carbs. Thus, alcohol slows down the fat-burning process. Second, alcohol contains 7 calories per gram, whereas carbs and protein both contain about 4 calories per gram, and fat contains 9 calories per gram. This means that alcohol is almost as bad for you as eating high-fat foods. And, once again, liquids don't satisfy you or fill you up.

In fact, alcohol does quite the opposite. Research has shown that alcohol not only decreases willpower, it increases appetite — specifically cravings for fatty and salty foods. Studies have shown as much as a 20 percent increase in calories consumed at a meal when alcohol was served beforehand. With the calories from the alcohol added in, there was a 33 percent total increase in calories.

Ray Audette, founder of the "Caveman Diet" in which dieters eat only what a prehistoric hunter-gatherer would eat (nuts, eggs, seafood and meat), confirms that alcohol works against anyone trying to burn fat and lose weight. Audette says, "Alcohol adds fat principally by producing cravings for both itself and other carbohydrates (see snack trays at any bar) and even other addictive substances (ask any former smoker.) It is almost impossible to drink alcohol and follow the hunter-gatherer lifestyle. If you must drink, do so only on special occasions (once or twice a year) and stick to alcohols derived from fruit (wine and champagne)."

While he also recommended abstaining from alcohol while dieting, the late founder of the Atkins diet, Robert C. Atkins, said, "If you must drink alcohol, wine is an acceptable addition. If wine does not suit your taste, straight liquor such as scotch, rye, vodka, and gin would be appropriate, as long as the mixer is sugarless; this means no juice, tonic water, or non-diet soda. Seltzer and diet soda are appropriate."

Truly, most people who have lost a great deal of weight and kept it off say that they gave up alcohol completely. If you do decide to keep alcohol in your diet, take Dr. Atkins's advice and stick to one glass of wine or low-calorie liquor, without a sugary mixer. Sorry, but margaritas are out.

Quit being clueless about what's in what you're drinking — it's just too easy to get hundreds of calories a day in liquid form. And remember that water is an easy zero-calorie alternative at any time.

Conclusion

Now that you've finished this book, there will be a lot of changes you'll want to start making right away. This can feel daunting and, truly, many weight-loss plans die before they even begin because people get overwhelmed and feel doomed to fail. Start by making a list of the main changes you want to make and bad habits you want to break, in order of priority.

Next, you'll have to determine whether you're the kind of person who feels better tackling the biggest issues first or the type who builds confidence from getting over the smaller hurdles first. Don't freak out or get burnt out. Some people benefit from a drastic lifestyle overhaul and others are baby-steps types. Take the "Ways to Lose Weight" in this book and actually make them work for you.

It is no small task to revamp your eating habits. The great thing about this book is that it doesn't make unrealistic demands of you, cut calories to the point that you're starving, or eliminate things that make you happy, such as eating out with good friends. Instead, it gives you options and alternatives, as well as the knowledge to make better, more informed food choices than you've been making. You can still join your colleagues at happy hour or eat a tasty breakfast, just without the guilt and weight gain. And the payoff will be when your friends and family notice your new choices and see the weight-loss results you're getting from them.

Pretty soon your new lifestyle will be your way of life and your bad habits will be a thing of the forgotten past. The next time you pick up this book, you'll say, "Wow, I can't believe I used to do that!"

Break your bad habits and embrace your weight-loss success, unbounded energy, and life at your new size and weight!

Additional Resources

Instant Diet Makeover covers the importance of redefining your food choices, creating a game plan to address each meal and craving, and making lifelong changes to your habits. This knowledge will definitely help you shed unwanted pounds; however, if try including exercise in your weight-loss program you increase the calories your body burns, thus propelling your weight loss even further. This section will give you additional information on complementing your new diet habits with a fitness and workout plan for amazing results.

Exercise to Jumpstart Weight Loss

A key element for weight-loss success is developing an exercise program. Choose activities that can be done each day so you can incorporate them into your daily routine. The length of time it takes to change from a sedentary to an active lifestyle can range from three weeks to three months. Get started by creating simple habits like walking more often when you're going somewhere in your neighborhood. Slowly add more exercises and increase the intensity as your body adjusts to each new activity.

So what is the best exercise regiment for you to embark on? The answer depends on your personality, interests, and individual abilities. The optimal solution is to choose an exercise program you will enjoy doing, and one that you will look forward to each day.

You have a wide range of options when creating a fitness plan. It can be slow, moderate, or physically challenging. You can do it all at one time, or integrate it into two or three segments over the course of your day. So build a physical activity plan that fits into your daily calendar, and keep in mind the common ingredient for any successful exercise program is to bring a measure of pleasure into it.

In addition to having fun and feeling energized, you will find that physical activity provides added perks, such as building muscle tone, curbing your appetite, and increasing your metabolism. One by-product built into a fitness-oriented lifestyle is improved overall health. It has been found that regular physical exercise reduces the risks of cancer, cardiovascular disease, and diabetes. It also provides psychological benefits, such as increased self-esteem and feelings of confidence. Getting more physically fit will have you feeling strong, mentally and physically, and will make you look great, too.

Creating a Physical Fitness Program

Your mission is to burn calories. Your new fitness program should include three essential elements for successful, long-term weight loss and maintenance: the first element is to include aerobic activities, which provide cardiovascular benefits; the second element is a resistance or strength-training program for improving muscle tone; and the third element is to consider integrating a basic stretching routine into your daily schedule to develop flexibility.

Before embarking on your mission, see a doctor to obtain a health clearance if you have unique health issues, injuries, or physical limitations. When you are ready to exercise, warm up slowly and be gentle on your body. It's the only one you've got, so take care of it as you work your way into top physical form.

Aerobic Activities: An aerobic activity is any type of body movement that speeds up your heart rate and breathing. It improves your ability to utilize oxygen, which increases your cardiovascular health. You can participate in aerobic activities almost anywhere: taking step classes at a gym, running in a park or riding a stationary bicycle in your home environment. The minimum amount of time for adult daily exercise is 30 minutes, and children benefit from 60 minutes per day. Keep in mind these numbers are a general estimate and should be tailored to fit individual needs. In all cases, use common sense when exercising and be sure to listen to your body. A general guideline for physical activity is to safely challenge your body while gradually stretching your limits.

Resistance & Strength Training: Once you have a personalized aerobic program that fits your style, consider adding a crucial piece of the puzzle to your fitness regime. Resistance and strength training will firm up muscles as the unwanted pounds melt away. This type of exercise should be done for 20 to 30 minutes, three times a week. It includes lifting handheld weights, using machines at a gym, or working out with videos in your home. If you choose to go to the gym, consult with professionals and learn how to correctly use the equipment.

Stretching & Flexibility: Stretching and flexibility are often neglected components of physical activity. Preparing the body for movement and keeping it injury-free should be built into every fitness program. Stretching and flexibility training is designed to develop range of motion, increase muscle elasticity, and achieve muscle balance. Stretching can also speed up recovery in preparation for the next fitness session. You should never stretch your body when it's cold or stiff. Be sure to start your physical activity with 10 to 15 minutes of slow movement until your muscles have warmed up. Mild stretching can be done at a midpoint in your daily training and again at the completion of the exercise program.

The best type of overall stretching routine is one that starts with the head and neck, working down toward the toes. It uses slow stretches that are held for a minimum of 10 seconds each. Avoid quick-pulling motions that put stress on muscles and joints. Choose abdominal exercises that support the lower back region. In all cases, consult with a professional for advice before beginning a strength and flexibility program.

Revamp Your Daily Routine to Include Fitness

If you are not the type of person who enjoys going to a gym, consider making your home environment a personalized recreational center. All forms of physical activity burn calories. So let's look at your daily chores in a new light: vacuuming for one hour burns 220 calories, grocery shopping requires 180 calories, and raking leaves expends 90 calories. If you have access to stairs, perhaps you might use them as your personal stair stepper. Walking up stairs in an easy and moderate manner for 15 minutes burns 120 calories.

Enjoy being outdoors? Try an afternoon of gardening, sweeping, raking leaves or mowing the lawn to tone up your arms, legs, and abdominals while you whittle away an additional 270 calories per hour. If you live in an area where it snows, you have hit the jackpot as shoveling snow consumes almost 600 calories per hour. Combining a few of these forms of aerobic activity is the equivalent of spending a couple of hours in the gym.

Incorporate Walking Daily

Perhaps home maintenance is not your idea of enjoyable exercise. Take a closer look at good old-fashioned walking. On a nice day, consider a stroll around your neighborhood. In cold or rainy weather, go to a local indoor mall and log miles while you glance at shoppers and window displays. This is a cost-effective activity that simply requires a good pair of walking shoes.

Walking may sound too good to be true, but it is an aerobic activity that burns calories. Consider the fact that walking at 2 mph, which is approximately a 30-minute mile, burns 200 calories. Walking a 20-minute mile at a

3 mph pace uses 240 calories. Walking a moderate, 15-minute mile, for an average of 4 mph, burns 300 calories. The faster you walk, the more calories you will burn.

Measuring a Mile: You may wonder how far you should walk to log one mile. After all, there are no standards when it comes to the length of suburban streets. There are a few methods of calculating distance. You can use a car to drive your neighborhood streets and look at your odometer to calculate mileage, or your may purchase a small pedometer to count your steps. The U.S. Surgeon General has recommended walking 30 minutes daily to strive toward a weekly goal of 10,000 steps, or roughly 5 miles. Those on a weight-loss program should strive for a minimum of 12,000 to 15,000 steps, which should take about 45 minutes per day.

Health Benefits of Physical Activity

Still need convincing that it is essential to change from a sedentary lifestyle to one that includes daily physical activity? Here are a few facts that might influence your decision: it has been found that regular physical activity reduces the risk of dying prematurely; exercise reduces the risk of developing heart disease, cancer, diabetes, and high blood pressure, and promotes psychological well-being. Exercise also helps decrease or eliminate depression and anxiety. Participating in physical activities is also an effective way to lose weight and maintain weight loss.

Exercise & Weight Control

Did you know that being overweight and being "overfat" are two different dilemmas? Some people, such as athletes, have a muscular physique and weigh more than average for their age and height. But their body composition, which is the amount of fat versus lean body mass (muscle, bone, organs and tissue), is within an acceptable range. Others can weigh within the range of U.S. guidelines, yet they can carry around too much fat. Use exercise as a way to balance your body fat percentage. An easy self-test is to pinch the thickness of fat at your waist and abdomen. If you can pinch more than an inch of fat, excluding muscles, chances are you have too much body fat.

Carrying around too much body fat is a nuisance. Many people fight the battle of the bulge through diet alone because exercise is not always convenient. Few of today's occupations require physical activity, and many people spend hours behind desks and computers. In addition, much of our leisure time is spent in sedentary pursuits. To reverse this trend, it is important to adjust your attitude and find time to exercise each day. Some of the most common reasons people use to avoid physical activity include:

1. "I don't have the time."
2. "I'm too tired and I don't feel like it."
3. "I'm not very good at exercising."
4. "It's not convenient to get to my workout place."
5. "I'm afraid and embarrassed."
6. "It's too expensive to join a gym."

Get out a journal and write down the reasons you've been avoiding exercise, joining a gym, or taking a fitness class. Now right down solutions to these reasons, which are really just excuses. For example, if your number one reason for skipping exercise is "I don't have time," you might consider taking half your lunch break to go for a walk or going for a bike ride with your family instead of going out for dinner.

There is *never* a good excuse to be sedentary. There are great gyms and fitness facilities of all types and price ranges. If you find the traditional gym environment isn't for you, try taking up a yoga or dance class. If money is a concern, sign up for a hiking club — things like hiking, swimming, rollerblading and biking are always free. The website MeetUp.com is great for finding groups of people with your similar interests in your area. And just look at how many ways there are to burn calories!

CALORIES BURNED FOR TYPICAL PHYSICAL ACTIVITIES

Light Activities: 150 or less	Cal/Hr.
Billiards	140
Lying down/sleeping	60
Office work	140
Sitting	80
Standing	100

Moderate Activities: 150-350	Cal/Hr.
Aerobic dancing	340
Ballroom dancing	210
Bicycling (5 mph)	170
Bowling	160
Canoeing (2.5 mph)	170
Dancing (social)	210
Gardening (moderate)	270
Golf (with cart)	180
Golf (without cart)	320
Grocery shopping	180
Horseback riding (sitting trot)	250

Moderate Activities: 150-350 (Cont.)   Cal/Hr.

Light housework/cleaning, etc.	250
Ping-pong	270
Swimming (20 yards/min)	290
Tennis (recreational doubles)	310
Vacuuming	220
Volleyball (recreational)	260
Walking (2 mph)	200
Walking (3 mph)	240
Walking (4 mph)	300

Vigorous Activities: 350 or More   Cal/Hr.

Aerobics (step)	440
Backpacking (10 lb load)	540
Badminton	450
Basketball (competitive)	660
Basketball (leisure)	390
Bicycling (10 mph)	375
Bicycling (13 mph)	600
Cross country skiing (leisurely)	460
Cross country skiing (moderate)	660
Hiking	460
Ice skating (9 mph)	384
Jogging (5 mph)	550
Jogging (6 mph)	690

Vigorous Activities: 350 or More (Cont.)	Cal/Hr.
Racquetball	620
Rollerblading	384
Rowing machine	540
Running (8 mph)	900
Scuba diving	570
Shoveling snow	580
Soccer	580
Spinning	650
Stair climber machine	480
Swimming (50 yards/min.)	680
Water aerobics	400
Water skiing	480
Weight training (30 sec. between sets)	760
Weight training (60 sec. between sets)	570

Your Workout Schedule

When creating your workout schedule, consider what you are trying to achieve. Since your primary goal is to lose weight and lose body fat, you will probably want to focus on cardiovascular activities, which burn fat and calories. However, your workout program should include all three components of fitness: cardiovascular conditioning, strength training, and flexibility. Working hard in all three areas will improve your performance in your target area. For instance, the more lean muscle mass you build, the faster you'll burn calories. A pound of muscle actually burns 3 times as many calories as a pound of fat. So get moving!

Another important aspect of each workout session is proper warm-up and cool-down activities. Be sure to include both of these in your program.

As you schedule your workouts for each week, be sure to take one day to rest. It's just as important to allow your body to recover and rebuild as it is to have a great workout. If you don't allow proper time for your body to heal and recuperate, you'll feel overtired, sapping your motivation to get off the couch and exercise. Take a day off here and there so you don't get burnt out.

If you are still unsure of where to begin, below are some activities that you should include in your workout program. Modify your workout program gradually as your endurance, strength and skill levels improve.

Warm-up: Begin with 5-10 minutes of low intensity/low impact exercise such as walking, slow jogging, knee lifts, arm circles, situps, or trunk rotations.

Strength training: Aim for at least two 30-minute sessions per week that may include free weights, weight machines, resistance equipment, muscular endurance training and toning activities such as Power yoga or Pilates. Focus on activities that exercise each of the major muscle groups or work more than one muscle group at the same time.

Cardio: Participate in a 30-minute session of aerobic activity at least three times a week. You want to make sure you're moving continuously and getting your heart rate up. You should be breathing hard at some point. Try a circuit training program that raises your heart rate and moves you quickly between activities or exercises. Typical activities include jogging/running, elliptical training, bicycling/spinning, and cardio classes such as step aerobics, kick boxing, and aerobic dance.

Flexibility training: Do 10-15 minutes of stretching per day. An easy way to incorporate flexibility training is by stretching for several minutes after your warm-up and during your cool-down. Yoga or Pilates are both fantastic workouts that also greatly increase flexibility and build fat-burning muscle.

Cool-down: Expect to take 5-10 minutes to cool down after your session. Your cool-down can include slow walking or low intensity or low impact exercises with your stretching.

Allow your heart rate, breathing and body temperature to gradually drop to normal levels. Use this time to relax and recover from your workout.

Water, Fitness & Weight Loss

Water is as essential to your diet makeover as it is to survival. Water constitutes more than two-thirds of the human body and is crucial to all of your body's major functions.

Maintaining hydration can have tremendous benefits for health and weight loss. Recent studies have shown that people who drink at least 8 glasses of water a day can decrease their risk of developing colon, bladder, and even breast cancer. And maintaining proper hydration keeps your metabolism working hard, maintains digestion, improves muscle tone, and makes your stomach feel full.

When to Drink Water

As important as it is to stay well hydrated, it's easy to forget to drink water until dehydration has already set in. Research has shown that the best time to drink water is before you feel thirsty. Physical signs like dry mouth and sensations of thirst often occur only after you are dehydrated.

The amount of water required for each individual is determined by his or her weight and metabolism. A rule of thumb for calculating your water consumption needs is to take your weight in pounds and divide it in half. The resulting number is the number of ounces of water you should consume. Some experts, however, suggest drinking even more water. They say that on average, men should drink around 120 ounces of water per day, while women should have around 90 ounces. No matter what your ideal water consumption is, remember to increase your water intake in conditions such as high heat, high altitude, low humidity, or high activity level.

Sources of Hydration

A number of liquids and solid foods can provide your body with the water it needs:

Water: Your body uses water most readily in its plain, unadulterated form. The bulk (80 to 90 percent) of your hydration should come from drinking plain water.

Beverages: Drinking non-caffeinated beverages, such as

low-calorie fruit juice and sports drinks and skim milk, is a good way of maintaining your hydration. Herbal teas also work well. Just remember to avoid beverages that contain sugar, fat, or both, which add unwanted calories to your diet.

Fruits and vegetables: Raw fruits and veggies consist mainly of water and are excellent for hydration. People who eat a healthy amount of fruits and vegetables may receive up to 20 percent of their hydration from these items.

Be wary of drinking caffeinated beverages, such as coffee, tea and many soft drinks. Caffeine is a diuretic, meaning that it stimulates your kidneys to remove water from your system. If you feel the need for a caffeinated beverage, remember to compensate by drinking extra water.

Hydration Before, During and After Your Workout

Proper hydration is one of the easiest and most effective ways of boosting workout performance. Water is necessary in order for metabolism to take place, so being properly hydrated helps your body turn food into the energy you need for exercising. Water also helps your body regulate its temperature through sweating. Because vigorous exercise causes you to lose large amounts of water through sweating, it is important to drink water before, during, and after each workout session.

Pre-workout: Drink between 8 and 16 ounces of water in the hour prior to working out.

During workout: Replenish fluids by drinking 4 to 8 ounces of water every fifteen minutes. During vigorous cardiovascular training, or if you're exercising in hot temperatures, increase your water consumption in order to replace water lost from sweating.

After workout: Drink between 8 and 16 ounces of water within thirty minutes of completing your exercise routine. Your muscles need water in order to recover from the stress of a workout. Drinking proper amounts of water after your workout will help reduce muscle soreness and help you feel less tired.

Since your goal is to lose weight, you should increase the amount of water you consume before and after working out. Water is necessary for metabolism to take place and keeps you feeling energized. Keep well hydrated to help your body burn calories and reach your weight-loss goals!